100 Ways to
Live
to 100

Also by Dr Roger Henderson:

Stressbeaters

100 Ways to
Live
to 100

How to Enjoy a Longer and Healthier Life

Dr Roger Henderson

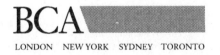

BCA

LONDON   NEW YORK   SYDNEY   TORONTO

This edition published 2002
by BCA
by arrangement with Judy Piatkus (Publishers) Ltd

CN 109064

Text design by Tracy Timson
Edited by Richard Dawes

Typeset by Palimpest Book Production
Polmont, Stirlingshire

Printed and bound in Great Britain by
Mackays of Chatham plc, Chatham, Kent

For my family

Acknowledgements

There are a number of people who should be thanked for helping with the writing of this book. My sincere thanks go to Judy Piatkus, Alan Brooke and Penny Phillips at Piatkus Books for being foolhardy enough to initially take me on and then polite enough to make encouraging noises as the book progressed. Mention should be given to Dr Ian Hoyle in Australia, whose reacquaintance with me after 17 years consisted of a number of medical queries out of the blue. Finally, I must mention my children – who continually remind me what is truly important in life – and my wife, with whom I hope to live to 100 and enjoy it!

Contents

Contents

Introduction

A century ago 60 would have been considered a fine old age, and anything over this something of an unexpected bonus. In 2002 the average lifespan for both sexes in the Western world hovers around 80, and the phrase 'three score years and ten', until recently used to denote a typical life expectancy, is now heard far less often. Indeed, the number of centenarians is increasing at a steady rate.

So why the change? What is it that has transformed us from a population dying at an age most of us now think of as late middle age, to one expecting to still be going strong well after 70? The answer is, as with so much of medicine, a combination of factors. Some of these are general points such as improvements in medicines and healthcare, sanitation and housing, whereas others are linked to lifestyle choice – what we eat, how we exercise, how conscientious we are about safety and how we now access health information more readily, to name but a few. All these factors and more have prolonged the ability of our bodies to tolerate the inevitable ravages of ageing that are programmed into every cell. Advances in medicine (especially in the field of genetics and disease screening) enable people who would otherwise have died much earlier not only to be kept alive but also to lead fruitful and enjoyable lives at the same time.

This touches on a key point, and one that I will return to repeatedly. This is not a book about trying to reach the age of 100 at any cost. Life is for living, and I see far too many patients who reach a point in their lives where – usually owing to infirmity – they are simply waiting for God. Living longer should always aim to involve enjoying rather than enduring, and I would personally choose to live a shorter and fruitful, happy life than a miserable one for the sake of reaching three figures. So, the point of writing this book is to try to show how the things under our control that actually affect our longevity can be altered for the better, allowing for an improved quality of life, rather than wasting energy on trying to change the things we cannot. A good example of this, and one I often see in my patients, is a slavish adherence to a low-fat diet while at the same time continuing to smoke or failing to take any kind of regular exercise. By focusing on one small risk factor (and one which has already caused damage long ago) such patients deny themselves one of the greatest pleasures in life – eating good food – even in moderation, become miserable as a result and, by ignoring other more significant risk factors in their life, do little to improve their overall health. There is nothing more dull in this world than a health bore, and a health bore following a slavish goal of living longer whatever the cost should be avoided at any price! I lead what I believe to be a healthy lifestyle – I do not smoke, I exercise regularly and in moderation (usually through a combination of walking my dogs and gardening – I gave up marathons years ago!), I watch what I eat and I keep my weight down. But I am no stranger to fish and chips, a drop of wine or standing on my head in the local swimming pool with my children. It is the pattern of our lives that affects our long-term health rather than the occasional fried meal or a drink or two – a point worth repeating often.

When talking about living long and healthy lives, we cannot ignore the degree to which luck can play a part. I am sure every reader can think of a distant Uncle Albert who daily smoked three packs of full-strength cigarettes and polished off a bottle of whisky, yet lived to be 106 before he was killed in a hang-gliding accident. Well, such freaks of nature do exist and always will. The problem, though, is that such people are trotted out as some form of scientific proof that smoking and heavy drinking do you no harm at all, and that 'it doesn't matter what you do in your life – just look at old Uncle Albert'. Such homilies are usually pronounced by the speaker with a degree of pride that suggests they feel the blessing of St Albert will keep them in rude health however they choose to live their life. Unfortunately, the Uncle Albert theory of old age falls down when it is realised that for every such rare anomaly in the laws of medicine, the remaining 99.9% of those attempting to mimic it have done the usual thing, followed the common rule of life and died prematurely.

Basically, there are three major factors that we can do nothing about and which may affect our ability to reach a ripe old age. The first is being male. Sorry, guys, but women do tend to live longer than men. The second is getting older. It's obvious really – as our bodies age the chances of something going wrong with them increase. Thirdly, family or genetic history plays a more crucial part in how long we live than most of us realise. Just as people whose parents and grandparents survived into their nineties or beyond tend to die at a more advanced age than the rest of the population, so those whose forebears die young appear to be less likely than most to live on and on. Fortunately, this principle is not carved in stone, but as a general rule it remains valid.

Incidentally, in writing about this topic, it seems sensible to consider those people who live the longest in the world and try to find out what they are doing right, and perhaps try to copy it. One such group inhabit the Japanese island of Okinawa. Later in the book I'll be looking in detail at some of the secrets of their remarkable longevity, but for the moment I'll leave you with an Okinawan saying: 'At 70 you are still a child, at 80 a young person. And if at 90 someone from heaven invites you over, tell him: "Just go away and come back when I am 100."'

I have chosen to split the book into five sections, offering twenty tips in each to give a broad view of the improvements that can occur by making simple changes in lifestyle or thinking.

These sections deal with medical factors, diet, lifestyle, natural treatments and the effect of the mind on the body. With each tip I have attempted to distil the current thinking and show its relevance to longevity, adding a brief 'takeaway tip' at the end for you to remember. You may be practising some of this advice already or may have never thought about your long-term health and be simply trusting to luck that you stay well. There is something for everyone here.

As a family doctor I have drawn on the everyday currency of my profession. The medical section is by no means exhaustive but covers the most important areas, as I see them in my daily work, you should pay attention to in order to maintain good health without too much trouble. I have approached the dietary tips in much the same spirit, and underlying them all is the belief that you do not have to be a nut cutlet-munching health fanatic who knits their own yoghurt to eat extremely healthily. The key is regular meals, eating fruit and vegetables every day and minimising the intake of refined foods, animal fats and sugar. A balanced diet contains all the five main nutrient groups in the correct proportions – proteins, carbohydrates, fats, vitamins and minerals. Feed your body junk and it will respond in kind. Give it the nutrients it craves and it will reward you by improving your health and general well-being.

Among the lifestyle tips are some that may not readily spring to mind. Do you know why flossing can improve your health? Why is sex recommended as a way of living longer? Can gardening be as healthy as running miles every day? The answers to these and many other questions are found in this section, and some may surprise you.

The inexorable rise in natural or alternative treatments shows how keen people of all ages are to seek more of a holistic solution to their health problems. This is why I have included a section on natural therapies as well as one on getting your mind and body to work together. With a growing body of evidence that natural treatments can also help patients, it is the ignorant doctor who sticks blindly to conventional medicine.

Forget the elixir of longer life – it simply does not exist. Instead, look at the crucial areas of diet, lifestyle, leisure activities and mental outlook, for here you will find the nuggets of gold that will make your life more fun and, yes, a lot longer.

'Ageing is bad, but consider the alternative.'

– Anonymous

Medical tips

Diabetes – the hidden iceberg

There are some medical conditions that, common as they are, become more apparent once you start looking for them. Top of my personal list of these undiagnosed illnesses is diabetes. Around 2% of the population of the Western world is diagnosed with the condition and there are probably just as many people unaware that they have it. Essentially, diabetes occurs when there is too much sugar in the blood, caused by the body having difficulty making enough of the sugar-controlling hormone insulin. There are two variations of diabetes, Type 1 and Type 2, both of which can shorten life.

Type 1, or insulin-dependent, diabetes is the less common, accounting for 10% of the cases of diabetes, and starts in childhood or early adulthood in half of these, before continuing throughout life. Type 2 diabetes, which forms the bulk of my diabetic workload, is more common in middle-aged and older people and more easily controlled with diet and tablets rather than insulin injections. The subtle difference between the two is that in Type 2 diabetes it is not a lack of insulin that is the problem but a resistance of the body's tissues to process insulin correctly.

One of the reasons why there are so many people with un-diagnosed diabetes (and in the UK a new case is diagnosed every ten minutes) is that there may be no symptoms at all, or a sufferer may simply become used to feeling tired and generally unwell. Classic symptoms include weight loss, tiredness, excessive thirst and drinking, and passing more urine than usual. There may also be persisting boils or infections that stubbornly refuse to clear up. All these symptoms tend to present more aggressively in Type 1 diabetics, who are usually diagnosed more rapidly as a result. In Type 2 diabetics, symptoms may be limited to excessive tiredness and so put down to 'old age' or 'getting old', which is very unfortunate since it is the work of a minute to check a patient's urine for sugar. If this is positive a blood test will usually confirm the diagnosis.

Treatment for Type 1 diabetes is insulin injections, which need to be given for life and may require a short stay in hospital, or specialist assessment to get the balance exactly right. In Type 2 diabetes, diet is usually the first-line treatment, with tablets or injections given only if this does not bring about an improvement after some time. For both types, vitally important is a good diet in which there is not too much sugar or fat and meals are regular. It is crucial to maintain an accurate control of diabetes, particularly as most Type 2 diabetics die of associated heart disease, often preceded by strokes, high blood pressure and impotence.

Dietary advice should always include eating less sugary and fried food, and more grilled food, roughage and vegetables. Many people forget how many calories are in alcohol and so undo all their good work with too many drinks each evening. Because of the risk of 'hypo' attacks, where the blood sugar falls too low as a result of missing meals or taking too much treatment, it is sensible to carry glucose tablets for emergencies as otherwise blackouts can occur. If these are happening you should contact your doctor since they suggest poor control of sugar levels. Do *not* stop insulin injections if you are unwell – a common mistake – and if you have any infections remember that these will affect diabetes adversely.

A rather chilling development in the seemingly relentless rise in diabetes has been the recent appearance of Type 2 diabetes in teenagers. Although this has already been recognised in America, it had never been seen in the UK before, and undoubtedly it reflects the high-fat, high-carbohydrate and low-exercise sedentary lifestyle of today's children and teenagers compared with those of 50 years ago. Gluttony really can be a deadly sin in such cases. Don't allow yourself to fall into the same trap.

Diabetes is one of the most common causes of shortened lifespan in the developed world. Watch out for the danger symptoms and get your sugar levels checked if you are worried. It really is better to be safe than sorry here.

Check your blood pressure

There are certain conditions that form the backbone of good health, and satisfactory blood pressure is one of them. If I measure one patient's blood pressure daily I must measure a dozen, and patients are often apprehensive to know if their blood pressure is all right even when there are no obvious reasons for them to worry. Basically, blood pressure is the pressure of the heart that forces blood around your body. This is not a constant pressure but varies throughout the day and night, being at its lowest when we are deeply asleep in the small hours and rising sharply during the first hour after waking. When blood pressure is consistently higher than normal throughout both day and night, the condition is called hypertension.

As blood pressure can be such a volatile measurement to take (and is often raised simply by going to the doctor to have it checked) I never view a patient as being hypertensive until I've taken a series of readings; a single reading is inadequate. If someone is found to be suffering from high blood pressure they are often surprised since, unless the readings are very high, most sufferers have no symptoms. Then I'm usually asked 'Why?', but in 90% of cases there is no specific answer – it just happens without an obvious medical problem being present, and this is known as primary, or essential, hypertension. In the remainder of cases the cause may be kidney problems, diabetes or certain drug treatments, but each is unique and needs to be investigated on its own merits.

In most cases of high blood pressure, and in the absence of other illnesses, the first thing you should do is alter your lifestyle. This always involves stopping smoking, losing weight if you are overweight and increasing the amount of exercise you take. The often forgotten keys to lowering blood pressure are to reduce dietary salt intake considerably, eat at least five portions of fresh fruit and vegetables each day and keep the intake of alcohol at approved levels. Finally, and often the most difficult of all, is to learn to slow down and relax more.

There is no doubt that the drug treatment of hypertension has been revolutionised over the past decade, and now often involves small doses of more than one drug to control blood pressure rather than very big doses of just one. This minimises side effects, and you should discuss the treatment of choice with your doctor. Recent large studies have shown few consistent or important differences in terms of the efficacy, side effects or quality of life between the different types of treatments currently available. It may be difficult for people to remember to consistently take their tablets when they are feeling well, but it is very important that they do so, because long-term control of blood pressure pays major dividends in reducing the risk of stroke, heart attack and kidney problems in later years.

When the blood pressure is well controlled, there should normally be a follow-up visit to the doctor every three to six months, but the American Heart Association has recently added another interesting fact into the melting pot. It now appears that bursts of stress such as occur in 'road rage' episodes and other aggressive outbursts may increase the risk of high blood pressure and heart attacks by three times that seen in more laid-back people. All the medical technology at our fingertips may therefore be no match for healthy doses of calmness and relaxation in our frenetic world!

High blood pressure is one of the biggest factors in poor long-term health. Know what yours is and act to bring it down if it is too high. Doing so will add years to your life as well as life to your years.

Think bones, think osteoporosis

I am a sucker for relatively useless statistics, and one I have recently come across is that every three minutes in the UK someone fractures a bone owing to osteoporosis. Thinning of the bones is an inevitable part of getting old, but when it becomes excessive it is known as osteoporosis, and such bones are more liable to break with injury. On average, women develop bone thinning about three times as quickly as men and this always worsens after the menopause, when the levels of the protective hormone oestrogen fall. By the age of 70, many women have lost a third of their bone, and although osteoporosis can happen at any age, about one in four women and one in 20 men will have fractured a bone as a result of this problem before the age of 65.

Although we are all potentially at risk of developing the condition, there are several key groups of people who are much more likely to do so than most. These include post-menopausal women not taking HRT (especially those who had an early menopause or a hysterectomy before it); people who have had prolonged periods of dieting or exercised to excess; and anyone who has been on high doses of steroids for many years. Others at high risk include smokers, heavy drinkers, women with infrequent periods for any reason and anyone who leads a couch-potato lifestyle with little or no exercise.

One of the problems here is that usually few, if any, symptoms are seen before a fracture occurs. The broken bone is usually the first thing anyone knows about their condition. Even minor falls or stumbles can cause serious fractures, and half of those who break a hip become unable to lead an independent life afterwards. There may be back pain owing to a fractured vertebra, or progressive loss of height and stooping – the so-called 'dowager's hump'.

With osteoporosis, prevention is always better than cure, simply because there is no cure, since once a bone is lost it cannot be replaced. But there is a great deal that can be done to improve the other bones and prevent further bone thinning. This includes regular exercise – even something as simple as walking will help – because the regular pulling by muscles and ligaments on the bones helps to stimulate bone-making cells and strengthen the bones. A diet rich in calcium is good, but if this is not possible, a daily calcium supplement may be taken. Every effort should be made to stop smoking, and excessive alcohol consumption avoided, although moderate drinking will do no harm. Hormone replacement therapy taken by women after the menopause will greatly reduce the chances of osteoporosis occurring. Ideally, this should be started within a year of finishing periods. However, if started at any time it will still cut down bone thinning but should be taken for five to ten years to achieve the maximum benefit for the bones. Other treatments include calcium and vitamin D tablets, and newer medication designed to strengthen bone, called biphosphonates.

Simply preventing falls is also a useful measure, and this can be as easy as checking vision and hearing, avoiding medication that causes drowsiness and making sure there are no trailing wires, slippery mats or treacherous floors in the house. On such small points a healthy – and long – life may depend.

Osteoporosis is a major cause of poor health and becomes more common the older we get. Reduce your risks by following a diet rich in calcium, stopping smoking and taking regular exercise.

Check your breasts

Until relatively recently there was a vogue among doctors for covertly checking women's breasts for lumps. In other words, if a woman presented with one set of symptoms the GP would try to check at the same time for breast cancer in an 'opportunistic screening' examination. Not surprisingly, this was not only deeply unpopular with many women – and rightly so – but on rare occasions over-popular with some unscrupulous doctors. Many of us breathed a sigh of relief when the UK's Chief Medical Officer of the day stated what we all knew: that it was inappropriate to perform routine breast checks on patients.

But breast screening remains something of a hot topic, especially as one woman in nine in the UK will develop breast cancer at some time in her life, and one woman in 11 in Australia, where there are 2,500 deaths annually. Each year just under 40,000 women in the UK are diagnosed with breast cancer and it is to our shame that this country has the highest mortality rate in the world for the disease. Although survival rates are slowly improving (mainly because of better breast awareness and improved drugs), over 13,000 women still die from this disease every year, of whom 1,200 are between the ages of 35 and 39. Four-fifths of breast cancers develop in women after the menopause and it claims more years of life from women under the age of 65 than coronary heart disease.

These figures are why the NHS has a breast screening programme that invites all women between 50 and 65 every three years for a mammogram – a type of X-ray that can detect abnormal breast lumps at an early stage and so increase the long-term prospects of that woman. (Men also get breast cancer but at a much lower rate – 200 or so cases annually.) The current government believes that screening for women under the age of 50 would not be of benefit, although trials are underway to see if this is incorrect, and women over 70 can – and, I believe, should – be screened, but they have to request this themselves. An overview of recent Swedish trials has shown that population screening across the age groups 40–69 is associated with a 21% reduction in breast cancer mortality. The Australian public health service allows one hour's paid leave every two years for cancer screening – important when one Australian woman dies from breast cancer every four hours.

It is hoped that the situation will continue to improve as a result of an increased awareness of screening, more experienced radiologists, better radiographic film and media promotion, but all this is no substitute for monthly self-examination. This and screening together provide the best way to detect any breast lump early, so if you are unclear about how to examine your breasts correctly, ask your doctor or practice nurse for more information. It really is worth one or two minutes of your time every month.

Breast cancer has a shocking mortality rate, and better self-examination and regular screening checks could prevent many deaths. Make sure you are familiar with how to examine your breasts, and if you are in doubt about any lump, ask, ask and ask again.

Have a smear

Cervical cancer remains one of the biggest killers of women in the UK, and it is a great tragedy that many of these women would still be alive today if they had had regular cervical smears. There are many reasons why women do not attend for regular screening – embarrassment and the fact that they feel well are two of the most common that I see – but there is good evidence that it may be saving one or two thousand lives each year. My back-of-envelope calculations show that we need to screen about 4,000 women to prevent one death. This may seem a somewhat labour-intensive method of screening, but the whole point is that while most abnormal smears are not cancers, they may well become so if left unidentified, and therefore screening is the best way to ensure this does not happen.

No test can ever be 100% reliable or foolproof, and since humans are analysing the cervical smears, errors can occur. However, these are much rarer than the tabloids would have you believe and there is even better news on the horizon. Scientists have now developed a test that – instead of looking for precancerous changes to cervical cells – checks for infection by the human papilloma virus (HPV), which has been linked to cervical cancer in more than 90% of cases. This test is almost error-free and is more likely to mean treatment is started early – a vital point when dealing with cervical cancer. The way HPV testing should be used would be to test women and then look for signs of persistent infection (these are what cause the most damage) by retesting, a year later, those women with a positive result.

So what's the problem? Well, unfortunately, many doctors have not heard of this test and even fewer women have. In the UK there is a nationwide pilot study involving over 10,000 women currently in progress to assess the efficacy of HPV screening, but in the meantime sexually active women from their early twenties to early middle age who are currently scrupulous about having smear tests may be less protected than they think. I can only hope that HPV testing becomes part of mainstream cervical cancer screening before too long, and there is also positive news for our paymasters too. According to HPV specialists, a combined HPV and cytology smear test would slice more than £30 million off the current annual cervical cancer screening bill of £130 million in the UK alone. Sensible whichever way you look at it.

Always make sure you are up to date with your cervical smears. These catch cervical cancer early and it is readily treatable when found in such cases.

Cholesterol – what's the fuss?

I have a theory about heart disease, but I doubt it will be found in any medical textbook. Let's call it Henderson's Law. You see, the Japanese eat very little fat, and suffer fewer heart attacks than the British, Americans or Australians. The French, however, eat a great deal of fat and cholesterol-rich foods and also suffer fewer heart attacks than the British, Americans or Australians. The Japanese drink far less red wine than the French, and suffer fewer heart attacks than the British, Americans or Australians, yet the Italians drink excessive quantities of red wine with the same result – fewer heart attacks. So there we have it. Conclusive proof that you can eat and drink what you like. It's speaking English that kills you. My Nobel Prize awaits.

When we talk about fat in our diets, we almost always mean cholesterol – a waxy substance that is made by our bodies because we need it to maintain the natural running of body cells. However, too much cholesterol in your blood can cause hardening of the arteries or atherosclerosis. And what does this cause? Heart attacks. Coronary heart disease (CHD) is one of the biggest killers in the UK, causing more than 135,000 deaths every year, and cholesterol is a major factor in this. Approximately 46% of CHD is caused by a total blood cholesterol of over 5.2 millimoles per litre and in almost every case it has been shown that reducing cholesterol levels reduces the risk of CHD. In fact, with a 10% reduction in cholesterol at the age of 40 the risk may be reduced by up to 50%, falling to 20% if it is reduced by this amount at the age of 70.

So, if you have a high cholesterol level and lower it, you can reduce or even reverse this build-up in the arteries and so lower your risk of illness or death from heart disease. Simple stuff, but it now becomes complicated by the fact that there is 'good' and 'bad' cholesterol, carried in the body by what are known as lipoproteins. Two types of lipoprotein affect your risk of heart disease, the first being low-density lipoproteins, or LDLs – the 'bad' cholesterol. LDLs carry most of the cholesterol in the blood, and the cholesterol and fat from LDLs are the main source of dangerous build-up and blockage in the arteries. So, the more LDL cholesterol you have in your blood, the higher the risk of heart disease. Then there are high-density lipoproteins, or HDLs – the 'good' cholesterol. HDLs carry some of the cholesterol in the blood, but this cholesterol goes back to the liver, which leads to its removal from the body. It can therefore be seen that HDLs help to keep cholesterol from building up in the walls of the arteries and hence reduce the risk of heart disease.

So far so good, but why should some people have too much cholesterol in their blood? Many factors are at play here, but key ones include:

★ Your genes. Heredity – what your parents passed on to you genetically – partly determines the amount of cholesterol your body makes, and I see many families where high blood cholesterol affects every person.

★ Diet. Obviously crucial, and highly significant given our fat-heavy Western diets. Saturated fats are found mostly in foods that come from animals and raise your cholesterol level more than anything else in our diet. Reducing the amounts of these fats is crucial in lowering blood cholesterol levels.

★ Obesity. Excess weight often increases blood cholesterol levels, so if you are overweight and have a high blood cholesterol, losing weight may help you to lower it.

★ Exercise. Lack of regular physical activity may help to raise LDL-cholesterol levels and to lower HDL-cholesterol levels. The opposite also applies, so exercise more to get LDL-cholesterol levels down.

★ Alcohol. This increases HDL-cholesterol, which is why we are so often told that 'red wine is good for you'. However, too much alcohol can damage the liver and heart, as well as causing other health problems, so always stick to recommended limits.

★ Stress. Now here's an old wives' tale. Over the long term, stress has *not* been shown to raise blood cholesterol levels. However, stress affects your habits and so many people, when stressed, eat fatty foods to comfort themselves. But it is probably the saturated fat and cholesterol in these foods that cause higher blood cholesterol, rather than the stress itself.

It is a good idea to get your doctor to check your cholesterol level if you do not know what it is, and, if it is raised, to do everything you are advised. This really is good medicine as far as your long-term health is concerned.

A high cholesterol level is a major factor in heart disease and sudden death. Get yours checked and take the appropriate action if it is raised.

Don't die of embarrassment

The French have their livers, the Americans their cholesterol levels and the British – well, the British have their bowels. I sometimes think that I could say anything to some patients, but as long as I have asked them how their bowels are they will be happy with what I tell them. Even so, many of us remain acutely embarrassed about discussing bowel-related problems. This might be amusing were it not for the fact that, in the UK, bowel cancer remains the second most common cancer in men and the third most common in women. Frustratingly for doctors, it is one of the most readily treated if found early enough, with 90% of early bowel cancers being curable. Recent surveys confirm our reluctance to think about bowel cancer, revealing that over half of people never look for blood before flushing the toilet, and fewer than one in four people recognise that bowel cancer can be a cause of persistent diarrhoea or bleeding from the bottom. Older people (aged 55 and over), however, are more likely to make this connection, which is fortunate as the majority of cases occur in this age group.

Common symptoms include a bowel pattern that is different from usual, bleeding from the back passage, weight loss and abdominal pain. The majority of cancers occur in the rectum and adjacent part of the large bowel. These can often be seen using a tool called a flexible sigmoidoscopy, which looks into the lower end of the bowel for small polyps, or growths, which are often the early signs of a developing cancer. Because polyps often grow slowly and painlessly, an increased awareness of the other symptoms to look out for is vitally important. Trials are currently underway to assess whether a single flexible sigmoidoscopy

17

examination at the age of 60 could be a safe and cost-effective way of cutting the number of deaths from bowel cancer. Initial findings show that 98% of people screened would not only have the test again but would recommend it to a friend. In addition, early figures reveal that one person in 300 screened has bowel cancer, which shows just how common this potentially curable disease is.

A strong family history of bowel cancer – such as parents or immediate relatives suffering from it – may indicate the need for screening to see if you are more at risk of this occurring. Fortunately, doctors are steadily accruing more information about the exact risks, which vary according to the closeness of the relative involved.

Bowel cancer is very common and very treatable. You will not make its symptoms go away by ignoring them. Get seen early, get treated early, get better quickly.

The prostate gland – where's that?

Many of the men who come to see me in my surgery do so for one of two reasons. The first is that they are concerned about their health, and the second is that they have been sent by their wife – often under protest – who is worried about them. One common such worry is about prostate cancer, usually following a media campaign highlighting the problem, and it is surprising just how poorly understood this cancer is, given that it affects one in 12 men during their lifetime. In the UK over 10,000 men die from it every year – one every hour – and the figure is only slightly lower in Australia. The tragedy is made worse by the fact that it is often readily treatable even when it has spread.

A hundred years ago the average life expectancy of a man in Europe or America was only 49. Now this figure is heading towards the 80 mark, and since prostate disease increases with age we will inevitably witness a steady increase in prostate cancer in the coming decades. Indeed, some estimates predict that cases of prostate cancer or benign prostate enlargement will double by the year 2020.

These statistics are due in part to the widespread ignorance there is about the prostate gland and why it exists in the first place. It is a small gland, about the size of a small walnut, that sits at the base of the bladder and whose function is purely to produce secretions to nourish sperm. It is normal for the gland to enlarge slowly during adult life, especially after the age of 50, which often gives rise to the symptoms described rather unkindly as 'old man's prostate'. The proper name for this condition is BPH (benign prostatic hypertrophy) and it is due to gradual pressure on or obstruction of the bladder as the prostate enlarges. Many of the resultant symptoms are similar to those of prostate cancer, although it is a completely unrelated condition.

The main symptoms of prostate cancer – in which prostate gland cells begin to divide and spread in an uncontrollable manner – are unique to each man, but there are several commonly recurring ones. Having to pass water frequently during the day or night, with a poor stream or dribbling, and having to wait for some time before being able to urinate are commonplace – and embarrassing for many men. There may be blood seen in the water, pain on urinating and occasionally back pain or impotence. Because prostate cancer is a slow-growing disease, it can be many years before it reaches a size where symptoms occur and it is diagnosed, although many men simply assume their problems are due to age and ignore them.

Although no one knows exactly what causes prostate cancer, we now have tests that are both simple and readily available which can detect the early stages of the disease and so make treatment easier. The first is a digital examination that allows the GP to feel the size, shape and texture of the gland. This is usually followed by a blood test known as a PSA (Prostate Specific Antigen) test, and a raised PSA level may call for an assessment by a specialist to see if any cancer cells are present. Ultrasound scans, biopsies of the gland and ordinary bone X-rays may all be taken to see if there is any tumour and whether it has spread outside the gland. Once this information is known, treatment may be commenced, although this needs to be tailored to the individual as there is no single course of action suitable for all patients. Examples of such treatments include surgery, radiotherapy, hormone therapy or no treatment at all. This latter choice may come as a surprise to many people, but in older men whose cancer is not aggressive or fast-growing this may be the preferred and safer option.

Know where the prostate gland is, what it does and what are the danger signs of prostate cancer. Cure depends on it being picked up early, so don't die of embarrassment.

Be wise – immunise

For the poet in me, autumn means a season of mists and mellow fruitfulness. For the doctor in me, however, it means one thing – flu. The UK influenza immunisation programme has steadily grown over many years to be a major health campaign that delivers over eight million doses of vaccine during a few weeks of each autumn, while in Australia the equivalent injections are available every April. Flu is a major killer every winter, and the vaccine has been shown unequivocally to reduce deaths from it as well as reducing hospital admissions and complications arising from it. In the last serious flu epidemic in the UK more than 30,000 people died, and most years this death toll remains at some 4,000 victims, mainly over the age of 65.

All of us have experienced flu at some time or other, but among the elderly and those with certain medical conditions – chronic heart, lung or kidney disease, diabetes or reduced body defences resulting from other medical treatments – the risk of serious consequences is considerable. More than any other illness, it is flu that causes the now seemingly annual 'NHS winter crisis' resulting from bed shortages, and patterns of deaths in winter closely follow the pattern of flu activity. The situation has recently improved slightly as far as vaccination is concerned, since otherwise fit people aged 65–74 are included for the first time in the 'at risk' group. Recent research into the efficacy of the flu jab in this age group has led to the recommendation that it should now be given routinely, and most health authorities in the UK have targets of at least 60% uptake each autumn among everyone aged over 65.

The vaccine is given as our 'best guess' as to which flu strains are going to reach each country every year, for it is acknowledged that flu viruses are able to mutate and change as they 'drift' across nations from year to year.

Many patients tell me they became ill with flu after immunisation and so are wary of having it again. Unfortunately, they are quite mistaken since there is no active virus in a flu vaccine and so it is a physical impossibility to catch flu from it. What may have happened is that flu was caught just before the vaccine was given, or another respiratory infection may have produced similar effects, but otherwise there is no problem here. Serious reactions to the injection are rare, although it can cause some discomfort and swelling at the site, as well as a temperature and aching muscles for a day or two. Food intolerance is not a sufficient reason for not giving the injection, although there are sometimes reactions in people who have a severe hypersensitivity to hen's eggs.

In the UK and Australia the vaccine is free to everyone (unless you choose to go to a private doctor or clinic). Immunisation really is a case of prevention being better than cure. Ask your doctor or practice nurse about being immunised, and whether you should also have a second immunisation, the pneumococcal vaccine, which prevents pneumonia in certain people such as those with heart disease and diabetes.

Flu kills and the elderly are most at risk. Prevent this by yearly immunisation; it's quick, free and painless.

HRT, Doctor – are you sure?

God is a man. The reason I can state this with absolute conviction is that if he was a woman he would have come up with a better blueprint for the menopause than he did. Now, I am no zealot when it comes to foisting hormone replacement therapy on to women whose menopausal symptoms are causing them undue misery, but I will say one thing. The art of being a good GP is being able to listen and not talk, and having listened to hundreds of women talking about HRT it seems to me that many of them have very high, almost unrealistic expectations about what it can do for them. Their decision as to whether or not they want to take it is usually influenced by media reports and talking to other women rather than by any hard clinical information. In the past I've often started a consultation about HRT with a patient who, as a result of being misinformed, would most likely stop taking her treatment if her high expectations were not met. Because of this I now make sure that I spend more time explaining the benefits of HRT to patients as well as talking about any fears and expectations they may have about it. I remind them that this type of treatment is, in effect, simply replacing hormones that they had naturally some years before. And I always try to include information about the long-term benefits, because if this is not discussed there may be only intermittent short-term use, which does not give any of the longer-term benefits for the heart and bones. My own view is that it should be continued for five to ten years after the age of 50 to get the maximum benefit from it.

As a firm rule, the only women who should avoid HRT are pregnant women, those with vaginal bleeding, cancer of the breast or womb, or severe liver disease. Any undiagnosed lumps in the pelvis must also be thoroughly investigated before treatment starts. Many women are surprised to learn that high blood pressure, blood clots or a history of fibroids of the womb need not prevent them from having HRT, although if any of these conditions is present their doctor will need to carry out very strict monitoring.

There seems to be a number of reasons why HRT is not taken by patients. The resumption of monthly bleeds is one that is often quoted to me, but this can be overcome by using the newer 'no-bleed' regimes, which appear to provide period-free HRT in up to 75% of cases. Another is a fear of cancer, especially breast cancer; the current thinking on this is that short-term HRT (up to five years) does not cause a significant increase in risk. After this time there may be some increase in risk, the degree of which is still being debated but which may be 12 cumulative excess cancers for every 1,000 users over 15 years' use. There is also a small but definite extra risk of blood clots and this needs to be discussed when thinking about HRT.

The overall benefits of HRT do seem to outweigh its risks, although it is not a magic cure-all. GPs and patients need to be in possession of all the facts, but if it is decided that HRT is the sensible option to take, the benefits are not just for the immediate problems. The risk of developing heart disease and osteoporosis are cut considerably, and there is now also evidence that some forms of dementia may be slowed if HRT has been taken in the past. As with so much of medicine, nutrition and herbal-based treatments are complementary factors here and should not be excluded or ignored but viewed as part of good medicine for the whole body.

HRT reduces the risks of cardiovascular disease and osteoporosis in later life. It is not a panacea, but you should discuss with your doctor what may be most suitable in your individual case.

Snoring, dangerous?
Never!

There is a question that I ask all my patients who have been recently involved in a road accident, and it's one that is guaranteed to raise their eyebrows: 'Do you snore?' This apparently nonsensical question is a very specific pointer to a condition which probably accounts for at least a third of all car crashes, possibly more where motorway driving is concerned – Obstructive Sleep Apnoea (OSA). It is more common in men than women, with around 4% of middle-aged men suffering from it, and it tends to peak around the age of 50. It is a condition where there is repeated obstruction of the airways through the night, with the result that the body wakes up time and again to try to clear this, although the sufferer will not be aware they are waking at all. There is never a chance to get deep, restful sleep and so daytime sleepiness, noticed especially when performing monotonous tasks or driving, becomes the norm. Some people are prone to this simply because of the way their upper airways are shaped, but most OSA sufferers are overweight and smoke or drink alcohol in the evenings. Other risk factors include conditions causing muscle weaknesses and the use of sleeping tablets.

Snoring is such a crucial factor in making the diagnosis that, in its absence, it is virtually impossible to say someone has OSA. The noise may reach heroic proportions, causing a partner to either sleep elsewhere or lie awake listening anxiously to long periods of silence that are suddenly broken by violent snores or gasps. Far from this problem being a music-hall joke, I have seen it destroy a number of marriages and this is partly why specialist assessment in sleep apnoea centres is often so important.

Simple measures may be enough to reduce the problem to

almost zero. Weight loss is the key one, but stopping smoking and drinking, reducing tranquilliser use and avoiding sleeping on the back are all important. Treatment is geared to the individual and based on investigations such as 'sleep studies', where the patient is monitored during sleep. Common solutions include the use of dental shields at night, surgery and continuous oxygen through the night to hold the airways open and so prevent apnoea attacks.

Although the UK and other developed countries are increasing, if slowly, the numbers of OSA specialists and clinics in recognition of the size of the problem, patients are often unaware of the link between their snoring and their chronic tiredness and so never present to their doctor for advice. A case perhaps of suffering in anything but silence.

Snoring is no joke if you have to listen to it, but the risks to the snorer could be more than you realise – and not just from their wide-awake partner! Sleep apnoea kills people. If you snore heavily and are constantly falling asleep during the day or when driving, see your doctor.

Get checked out

It is no more than common sense to realise that by performing self-examination and having regular medical check-ups you not only improve the chances of early detection of a problem but also increase the possibility of making a full recovery from any illness that is discovered. Many people, however, do not do this, either because they do not know what they should be looking for or because they take a more fatalistic 'wait and see if it happens to me' approach. Unfortunately, even though it is a simple thing to get checked out occasionally, we probably spend more time pondering what lottery ticket numbers to pick than thinking about regular health checks.

Both men and women should check their skin regularly for new growths, such as sores that do not heal or moles that change in size, shape or colour. Warning signs like these should be reported to the doctor right away.

Don't forget your dentist for health checks – they should examine your mouth at regular intervals. In between visits use a mirror to check inside your mouth for changes in the colour of the lips, gums, tongue or inner cheeks, and for scabs, cracks, sores, white patches, swelling or bleeding. If you have any such symptoms, these need checking, especially if you are a heavy drinker or smoker, or are over the age of 50.

Men should always be aware of possible prostate problems and in an ideal world should have a regular digital rectal examination to check the prostate for hard or lumpy areas. However, this is contentious and is far more aggressively promoted in America than in the UK, but as part of a general 'well man' check it should always be discussed and performed if appropriate.

Whereas prostate cancer is the domain of the middle-aged and older man, testicular cancer occurs most often between the ages

of 15 and 34. Most of these cancers are found by men themselves, often by doing a testicular self-examination, or by their
partner during lovemaking. If you find a lump or notice another
change, such as heaviness, swelling, unusual tenderness or pain,
you should see your doctor.

For women, breast screening is discussed earlier in this section of the book, but it's worth repeating that the sooner any
breast cancer is found the more treatment choices that woman
has and the greater her chances of complete recovery. It is therefore vital that the condition is detected as early as possible. A
woman should talk to her doctor about it, especially if there is
a family history of breast cancer, ask about the symptoms to
watch for and establish an appropriate schedule of check-ups.
She should also ask about mammograms (X-rays of the breast),
well-woman health checks and breast self-examination (BSE).
By doing BSE, a woman learns what looks and feels normal for
her breasts, and is more likely to detect any change. Fortunately,
most breast lumps are not cancer, but it is always important to
have a breast lump examined as soon as possible.

Regular smear tests are designed to detect early cancer of the
cervix, and here a sample of cells is collected from the upper
vagina and cervix with a small brush or a flat wooden stick. The
sample is placed on a glass slide and checked under a microscope
for cancer or other abnormal cells. Smears should begin in women
when they turn 18 or become sexually active and although cervical screening will never prevent all cervical cancer there is good
evidence that it is saving 1,000–2,000 lives a year in the UK
alone.

Regular checks are not infallible, since they only give a snap-
shot of how someone is on that particular day. However, it is far
better to be looking out for early illness than not – just ask my
patients who have had their potentially serious problems picked
up early in this way.

Know what kind of self-examination is useful and how often to do it. Your doctor or practice nurse will help you with this. And although regular check-ups with your doctor may be an inaccurate science, they are far better than none at all.

Keep taking the tablets

Occasionally I get a major belly laugh from my work. One of the most recent examples of this was when a very pleasant chap came back to me complaining that I hadn't prescribed his normal tablets. On checking my computer I found that, although the supplier had changed, his actual tablets had not, and I queried why he believed this to be so. 'Well,' he said, 'the other lot always used to sink when I put them down the toilet. This lot float.'

It's not often this extreme, but non-compliance with doctors' instructions about medication is a major problem and one of the reasons they always tell their patients to 'finish the course of treatment'. Although hard facts are a little tricky to come by, for obvious reasons, it has been estimated that at least 50% of patients fail to comply with drug therapy for chronic conditions, and I have no problem at all with believing this figure to be correct. Poor compliance is undoubtedly the main cause of non-response to medication and is obviously dangerous, causing significant morbidity and mortality. Talking to other family doctors, I've found that there seems to be an accepted 'rule of thirds' where treatment is concerned. One third of people probably take their medication correctly, one third take some and then forget to take the rest and one third don't even bother to hand in their prescriptions to the pharmacist or, if they do, don't take the drugs. Knowing this, one of the things I often do on home visits is try to look in a patient's bathroom cabinet, and I am commonly assaulted by months of unopened boxes of pills pouring out on to the floor.

In America, where figures on this problem are slightly more readily available, it is called the world's 'other drug problem' and is said to cause over 100,000 deaths annually, with 10% of all hospital admissions being linked to non-compliance with treatment. It is likely that these figures correlate with findings in the UK and other countries, so why should there be such a problem with taking tablets?

Medication non-compliance – defined as the failure to take drugs on time in the dosages prescribed – has many causes. I believe many patients leave my surgery and then weigh up what I have told them against their own perceptions of risk and benefit and decide against treatment. If they do not believe themselves to have a major problem – for example, patients with high blood pressure but no symptoms and who feel well – then they see no need for regular daily treatment. Side effects, or the belief that side effects will be major once they have read the drug information that now comes with all prescribed medication – a major *bête noire* with me – is another common factor.

Patients whose doctors take the time and trouble to explain why a medicine is being prescribed, what its effects and side effects are, and how long it needs to be taken for are much more likely to comply with treatment than someone who has a prescription shoved under their nose and is told to go away and take the tablets. With the time pressure on GPs so severe nowadays, giving this information to a patient is sometimes sacrificed, and so it behoves us all to remember that medication actually needs to be taken to work!

Always take any medication as prescribed. If you have any concerns about why you are taking a particular treatment or simply want to know more about your prescription, ask your doctor or pharmacist.

Remember Medic Alert

Picture the scene – you are walking along the street when, without warning, you collapse. This could be due to an existing medical condition you are aware of, or it might simply have struck out of the blue even though you were previously fit and well. Without being able to ask you, how many clues can passers-by or attending paramedics find to work out what has happened? Usually the answer is none, which often leads to a crucial delay in diagnosis and treatment that may make all the difference between life and death. Many lives have been lost in this way, and relevant here is a recent rise in deaths attributable to severe allergies and ana-phylactic shock, such as occurs in full-blown peanut allergy. The tragedy is that some of these fatalities probably could have been avoided by one of the lowest-tech items anyone could use – a simple bracelet.

The Medic Alert Foundation produces bracelets and necklets engraved with the particular condition of the wearer for situations where they are unable to speak for themselves, such as an accident or a medical loss of consciousness. Also engraved on the device are a personal identification number and a 24-hour emergency telephone number. The use of this information need not be restricted to the country of issue, since should an emergency occur abroad the wearer's medical details can be relayed to medical personnel anywhere across the globe. There is also the extra advantage of designated family and friends being notified about any crisis, as well as physician follow-up being available.

Like many outstanding ideas, the whole concept of Medic Alert bracelets grew out of a relatively minor incident. In 1956 an American teenager cut her finger while playing and was taken to hospital by a neighbour since her parents were away that day. In the course of treatment she was given a routine sensitivity test to the horse serum used in a tetanus antitoxin and immediately developed a massive allergic reaction to the serum. After being critically ill for some days she fortunately recovered, but her father, a doctor himself, began to wonder about ways to prevent any such incident occurring again. The result was a bracelet, worn by his daughter, with all her vital medical information and allergies detailed on it. This idea rapidly spread and there are now some four million people throughout the world who belong to the Foundation. In the UK there are nearly 200,000 members and some 9,000 new applications annually, with all participants identifiable by carrying the familiar bright-red 'serpent and staff' insignia of the medical profession. The 24-hour emergency telephone line is manned by staff with medical knowledge who can supply emergency services with any required information instantly, and such speed is vital in cases where minutes can make all the difference.

Endorsed in the UK by the Royal College of Physicians and the Royal College of General Practitioners, as well as by many other medical societies, Medic Alert, which is a registered charity, has proved its worth time and again over recent years and thousands of people now owe their lives to its existence. The system is also widely in use in Australia.

As part of the only medically validated emergency system currently available, Medic Alert's identification tag is perhaps the only example of a designer bracelet worth more than its weight in gold.

Who needs Medic Alert?

★ Anyone with a medical condition that may be life-threatening.

★ Anyone with diabetes, a tendency to seizures or Alzheimer's disease.

★ People reliant on specific and regular medications.

★ Organ-transplant patients.

★ People with severe allergies to certain foods, medication or insect bites.

★ People with severe medical conditions that may not be immediately apparent.

Sun, sea and skin cancer

One of the less appealing qualities of the British is their predilection for exposing vast expanses of white flesh to the sun whenever we actually get good weather. On a Monday morning after a sunny weekend I'm always having to deal with many cases of severe sunburn, often in young children as well as adults. As our understanding of skin cancer grows, however, the idea of a tan being good for you looks increasingly like a sick joke. Rather more worrying is the fact that in a recent survey less than 50% of patients linked skin cancer with sun exposure. When you add foreign travel, sunbed use and the poor old ozone layer to the equation, it is little wonder that the number of cases of skin cancer is rapidly increasing to over 40,000 per year in the UK, while the figures are even higher, relative to population size, in Australia.

The most dangerous form of this condition is the malignant melanoma. These are commonest in women and people with fair skin and blonde or red hair, although anyone is at risk of developing them. There is now good evidence that sunburn occurring before the age of 16 also increases the risk of melanomas in later life, so advice about sensible protection from the sun should begin at an early age. This includes avoiding the midday sun, when exposure to light of the damaging ultraviolet-B wavelength is at its greatest; wearing cloth caps and hats (if you hold clothing or hats up to sunlight and you can see sunlight through them, they offer little protection); and using high-factor sun block whenever possible, rather than 'tanning' creams. With proper precautions and education from a young age – such as the 'no cap, no play' rule in Australian schools – the incidence of melanomas should fall in the coming decades. However, this is of little comfort to my patients who are currently suffering from this disease, all of whom enjoyed long days tanning themselves in pursuit of the body beautiful but whose bodies are now tragically anything but.

It is worth remembering the 'ABCD' rule about skin moles and the danger signs to look for. Is there any Asymmetry to the mole? Does it Bleed? Has it changed Colour or gone dark or black? Is its Diameter increasing in size? If the answer to any of these questions is yes, a medical opinion should be sought. Doctors would much rather give reassurance about a harmless mole than see a malignant melanoma too late in the day to be able to help.

Patients with melanomas often tell me with some bitterness that there is no such thing as a safe suntan. Indeed, one recently commented, 'Whoever said beauty is only skin-deep sure got it right.' Unfortunately, they were.

Skin melanomas are readily preventable. Keep your exposure to the sun sensible, remember the 'ABCD' rule about moles and never make the mistake of thinking that tanned skin is healthy skin.

Keep the winter blues away

If I were to ask 100 of my patients chosen at random how they feel in general during the long, dark nights of winter, a great many would say 'a bit depressed'. They are nearer the truth than they realise, since many people feel low at this time of year. The phenomenon was recorded as far back as 430 BC by Hippocrates, and although he did not give the condition a name, we call it seasonal affective disorder (SAD). Exactly how common this appears is unclear, but the SAD Association in the UK suggests that around one million Britons experience significant winter depression, with another ten million getting a milder form of 'winter blues'. Figures for Australia are proportionately the same. These are huge numbers, and although they cannot be strictly validated, what is certain is that many people in both countries and others throughout the world suffer from a clinical depressive illness during the winter but not at other times of the year.

If I am considering this diagnosis, I look for evidence of cycles of definite clinical depression over at least three consecutive years as it is the pattern of someone's behaviour over this time rather than during seasons taken in isolation that is important. There is usually tiredness, lack of motivation and sometimes weight loss, as well as an altered sleep pattern. Suicidal thoughts are seen less commonly in SAD than in other forms of depressive illness, but this becomes more of a risk if the depression worsens.

Treatment varies. Pure clinical depression should be treated conventionally with antidepressants, chosen to suit that particular individual, and I have also had great success with the natural herbal treatment St John's Wort, or hypericum. (This can be bought without a prescription, but ask your doctor's advice before using it.) For most people, however, therapy is simpler – light. It is believed that SAD arises from a lack of daylight (and possibly sunshine), which reduces production of the brain chemical serotonin. Using light boxes to stimulate the natural production of serotonin does seem to help certain patients, and these are used in large numbers in Scandinavia. They are *not* sunbeds, goggles are not needed and normal activity can continue around them. Two weeks is often enough to bring about an improvement.

SAD blights many people's lives, but because it often goes unrecognised it causes misery when it need not. Many sufferers are surprised when I suggest light therapy, but this works, and works well – try it and see.

Winter blues can be severe and debilitating. Avoid dreading each winter by using the oldest treatment there is – light.

Know about ovarian cancer

Some of the illnesses that I see in my job I hate simply because of the effect they have on the lives of my patients. Near the top of my personal hit list is ovarian cancer, which is among the five most prevalent cancers in the developed world. It is the fourth most common cancer in the UK, where nearly 7,000 cases occur each year. In Australia over 1,000 cases are diagnosed annually and there are some 800 deaths from the disease. For this cancer there are currently no screening tests recommended for the general population, although clinical trials are ongoing in order to determine whether screening would be cost-effective.

Risk factors for ovarian cancer include the commonest one of the lot – age. Half of all cases occur after the age of 65 and most are after the menopause. If there is a strong family history of ovarian, breast or bowel cancer, the risk may increase, but inherited ovarian cancer remains relatively rare. Genetic factors include the inheritance of genes known as BRCA1 and BRCA2 and in some ethnic groups, such as Ashkenazi Jews, up to 30% of ovarian cancers may be inherited. If a woman has never been pregnant, then her risk is higher, as is that for any woman with a history of breast cancer, but factors that appear to reduce the risk include taking the contraceptive pill and breast feeding.

I get especially angry with ovarian cancer because it is so insidious and I often see cases that have become quite advanced before the diagnosis can be made. This is partly because in its early stages it often has few, if any, symptoms, and when they do occur they can be so vague as to not clearly suggest the condition. These include swelling of the abdomen that does not go down, abdominal pain or discomfort, digestive problems, weight loss and a frequent need to pass water.

Diagnosis requires a combination of abdominal ultrasound scans, blood tests, X-ray of the kidneys and using a 'keyhole' fibre-optic camera called a laparoscope to look inside the abdomen directly at the ovaries. Treatment, which depends on the stage the cancer has reached, includes surgery, chemotherapy and radio-therapy. However, early recognition of symptoms obviously speeds up both the diagnosis and treatment of the condition. So, if just one woman reading this book recognises her symptoms as being similar to those described here and consequently has her ovarian cancer – which would otherwise kill her – picked up at an early stage, then I will be a very happy man indeed.

Ovarian cancer is often a silent killer because people are unaware of its symptoms. Always ask your doctor's advice about it, even if you are worried you might be making a fuss over nothing. There is no room for pride in the grave.

Beware of depression

For a condition that affects at least one in five people at some time in their life, there is a great deal of misunderstanding surrounding depression. This is a clinical illness that can strike – sometimes with great speed – anyone, at any time and at any age. It does not mean a sufferer is going mad (a common myth) or that they are going to somehow 'pass on' their depression to other people. This would be laughable if it were not a serious belief in some families I look after.

Depression often presents as overwhelming feelings of despair, hopelessness and helplessness in the face of everyday activities. It causes both psychological and physical symptoms, including very real physical pain. Spike Milligan – one of the famous sufferers from the illness, along with Winston Churchill and Florence Nightingale – described very eloquently his dread of his depression returning because of the amount of pain he knew he would be in.

Although both men and women become depressed, in my experience men are more likely to throw themselves into hard work, hard drinking, hard exercise or hard fighting to try to 'pull themselves out of it'. However, as I often say to my depressed patients, you can no more pull yourself out of a full-blown clinical depression than you can pull yourself out of a broken leg. Often triggered by a life event such as bereavement, serious illness or the loss of a job, it can occur without warning. But it can have an inherited element, so that a strong family history of depression may make you slightly more likely than others to suffer from it at some time.

The symptoms vary widely, but common psychological ones include despair, over-sensitivity, self-hatred, feelings of guilt and lack of motivation for any task. Physical symptoms include weight loss, loss of sex drive, insomnia, forgetfulness, restlessness and physical aches and pains. In severe depression there may be thoughts of suicide, failure to eat or drink and even hallucinations or delusions.

Treatment is available and very effective, although there is often a barrier to success in the depressed person's reluctance to admit to having a problem. Antidepressant tablets remain the commonest way GPs treat depression, but many (including me) have been guilty of stopping taking these before a full recovery has been effected. Because many cases of depression appear to be linked to low levels of certain chemicals in the brain, drug treatment is often aimed at boosting these levels and so easing the symptoms. Unfortunately, not only can antidepressants have significant side effects but there is also a significant relapse rate when they are stopped. However, when they are combined with cognitive behavioural therapy (CBT) the results are much better. CBT is essentially a way of changing how you feel by changing the way you think. It helps you to stamp out negative thinking and encourages you to take control of your own thought patterns. CBT has also been shown to be effective at treating many other mental disorders, but if your doctor has not suggested this type of treatment to you, there is probably a very simple reason – there are relatively few such therapists available on the NHS.

Depression kills people, often at a tragically early age. Never be afraid to admit to feelings of depression, as it is far more dangerous to ignore them and hope they will go away.

Understand asthma

Asthma is a problem with breathing caused by a narrowing of the airways through which air moves in and out of the lungs. Among children it is the commonest lung condition, and the number of sufferers – both children and adults – is increasing. As many as 1 in 15 adults in the UK suffers from asthma, and in England and Scotland alone about 1,500 deaths from the disease occur every year. The figures are not much better in Australia, where the average mortality rate over the past five years is 460.

The cause of asthma remains unknown, and many things appear to bring on attacks, including allergies, pollution (which may explain why asthma continues to increase) and emotions. Other things known to trigger asthma include:

★ pregnancy

★ cold air

★ cigarette smoke, perfumes and chemical fumes

★ pet hair

★ medication such as aspirin, beta-blockers and anti-inflammatory drugs

★ exercise.

Asthma attacks tend to occur intermittently, every few days, weeks or months, depending on the severity of the condition. Coughing and waking at night are common, but many sufferers take these problems for granted and do not mention them to their doctor.

Wheezing is often worse early in the morning or on waking and the classical asthma attacks that I see involve a sudden shortness of breath, wheezing and coughing. The chest feels tight and the patient may panic that they are going to stop breathing. More severe attacks may cause patients to lean forward and put their arms on their knees to try to get more air. They may only be able to speak in gasps, saying a few words at a time. During a severe attack the quieter the patient becomes the more I worry.

Treatment depends very much on the type of asthma and how severe the attacks are, but it is generally one of two types. The first is everyday treatment to prevent attacks and allow for a normal quality of life; this is known as preventive, or prophylactic, treatment. Two main types of drug are used here, given usually as inhaled treatment, which is preferred to tablets or liquid medicines. There are 'preventers', which are inhaled steroids taken on a regular basis to reduce any inflammation in the airways that may cause symptoms of asthma. Secondly, there are 'relievers', which have a much shorter length of action and are used to immediately relieve symptoms. These medications are also inhaled, and, because they act directly on the surfaces of the airways, any absorption of the drug into the rest of the body is minimal. If asthma proves to be poorly controlled, other treatment can be added to the usual inhalers. This includes other kinds of inhalers and tablets. Excessive use of the 'reliever' inhaler during the day or night suggests that either more 'preventer' is needed on a regular basis or extra treatment needs to be added to what is being taken.

If emergency treatment is needed, the aim is always to open up the airways as quickly as possible and so relieve the symptoms. The quickest way to do this is to give reliever medication through a nebuliser. This hand-held device, powered either by battery or mains electricity, produces a very fine mist of the drug dissolved in water which is then breathed in through a mask held to the face. In most cases this begins to relieve the symptoms within minutes. But if symptoms persist, oxygen may be needed and it may also be necessary to admit the patient to hospital, where injectable treatment can be given under close supervision.

The aim of asthma treatment is to ensure that the condition does not reduce the patient's quality of life, and indeed most sufferers are able to live normally. Increasing the use of preventer and reliever inhalers, sometimes with the addition of antibiotics if a chest infection is present, can stop most attacks. For more persistent attacks, nebulised treatment or steroid tablets may be needed, but if the condition is not responding to the patient's usual treatment it is important to seek medical advice promptly.

After a time many asthmatics are able to work out what tends to bring on their attacks. Once you have identified these triggers – for example, dust, cigarette smoke and any foods which appear to make things worse – the best treatment is to avoid them, as well as taking regular preventive medication. Regular, steady exercise – especially swimming – has a beneficial long-term effect, although sudden exertion can sometimes trigger an attack. Smoking should be stopped immediately. Make sure you are not taking medication such as aspirin, beta-blockers or non-steroidal anti-inflammatory drugs used to treat arthritis and similar conditions. If you are prone to bad attacks of stomach acid (also known as acid reflux), where the acid comes up into the gullet, reduce the risk of this, since it can trigger airway irritation, by losing weight, cutting down on coffee and alcohol and eating a sensible diet. If stress appears to make your asthma worse, try to keep your stress levels to a minimum whenever possible.

Here endeth the brief lesson on asthma. I still hear of too many deaths from asthma, often at a young age, and what is particularly sad is that a large number of these could have been prevented by the correct treatment or better understanding of the condition by the patient. We owe it to asthma sufferers to try to make sure that such tragedies become a rarity.

If you have asthma, make sure that you not only understand what causes it but also what your treatment is designed to do and how it should be taken. Even if you are feeling well, do not be tempted to simply stop or alter your treatment. Always check with your doctor or asthma nurse first.

Watch out for danger symptoms

I have a cartoon at home which shows a GP standing beside the bed of a worried-looking patient. Next to him stand a smartly dressed consultant and a smiling chap in a Hawaiian shirt and shorts. The GP is saying to his patient, 'I've taken the liberty of calling in a second opinion. One is a consultant, the other is an enthusiastic amateur.'

What would distinguish the approaches of these two medically interested types? The main difference would probably be that if the amateur were asked to list danger symptoms in the patient he might get three or four and then dry up, whereas the consultant would probably still be going at around the 20 mark. The question, 'So what symptoms should I be looking out for, Doc?' is one I hear more often than you might think. Now, although any list of symptoms is far from likely to be exhaustive, there is a common list that I think is worth giving here. I shall call it 'Henderson's Top Ten'. In no particular order (and excluding the one everybody is aware of – chest pain), these symptoms are:

★ Tiredness. Profound or prolonged tiredness that cannot be explained by a lack of sleep or other simple problem should be investigated. Fortunately, the vast majority of 'TATT' (tired all the time) patients have no serious illness, but if they did I would last about a week in my job as it is so common a symptom. However, if the tiredness is different from normal it should be checked out.

★ Weight loss. Sudden or unexplained weight loss should *always* be investigated. Whereas weight gain is rarely a sign of sinister problems, unexpected weight loss can sometimes be the first sign of serious illness somewhere in the body.

★ Easy bruising. If simple knocks or bumps cause severe bruising, a blood test may be needed to check all is well. Although the skin and blood vessels become more fragile with age – and many elderly people bruise very easily as a result – if there is significant bruising (especially if the gums bleed too) for no obvious reason, this should be investigated.

★ Trouble swallowing. Simple acid reflux into the gullet can cause this, but any difficulty in swallowing food – especially bread or meat – that develops over any length of time may not be due to a benign problem. If there is difficulty swallowing liquids, a doctor should be consulted as soon as possible.

★ Rectal bleeding. Bleeding from the back passage should never be ignored as being due to 'piles'. Although haemorrhoids remain the commonest cause of such bleeding, never assume this is the case without getting it confirmed by your doctor. The reason for doing so is that another disease may also be present, such as bowel cancer, and, as any doctor will tell you, 'If you don't put your finger in it, you'll put your foot in it!' Bowel cancer is sometimes allied to the following condition.

★ A change in bowel habit. Although we all have days when our bowels are not as regular as usual, any change in pattern lasting more than a fortnight should be assessed. This could be unexplained diarrhoea, a feeling that the bowels have not emptied properly in some way, the sensation of wanting to go to the toilet again immediately, or becoming constipated unexpectedly.

★ Blood in the urine. Known as haematuria, this is sometimes due to water infections but can be a sign of bladder growths. Even if there is no pain with the bleeding, always take a water sample to your GP and get it checked.

★ Headaches. Everyone gets headaches from time to time and the usual cause is tiredness, stress or poor posture. But you should never ignore headaches that refuse to go with painkillers, or are chronic, or are associated with nausea, vomiting or blurred vision, or that wake you.

★ Unusual vaginal bleeding. Any woman who has unexpected bleeding after the menopause, or has bleeding after intercourse, should be examined. While there are many benign causes for this problem, there are also a number of worrying ones, and if you are in doubt always get yourself checked.

★ Jaundice. Yellow discoloration of the eyes and skin is never normal and must always be assessed. This symptom can be due to a number of problems, ranging from the relatively harmless to the serious, the latter including viral infections of the liver, cirrhosis and tumours.

In each case the bottom line remains the same. If you are worried about a health problem, see your doctor. That's what we're there for.

If you are not sure whether a symptom could be serious, always ask your doctor. It may be the most important question you ever ask in your life.

'Anyone can get old.
All you have to do
is live long enough.'

— Groucho Marx

Diet tips

Coffee in moderation

I am fond of looking at old cartoons and the magazine *Punch* has had some brilliant ones in its pages. One of my favourites is from a century ago: a disgruntled member of a gentlemen's club is addressing a waiter, saying, 'Look here, Steward, if this is coffee, I want tea; but if this is tea I wish for coffee.'

Caffeine leaves me somewhat equivocal as far as health is concerned, yet it remains one of the best-researched substances in the food industry. It has no nutritional value, is not required by our bodies physiologically and is heavily abused by the tired and stressed. For these reasons health gurus often roundly condemn it, but the vast majority of the medical evidence currently available suggests that in moderation it has no adverse effects on our long-term health. So why should I be mentioning it at all in this book? Well, because many heavy coffee drinkers do other things that are not conducive to good health. Surveys show that they are also more likely to smoke, eat a high-fat diet and exercise infrequently, if at all. (In case you were wondering, tea drinkers tend to exercise more and eat more fresh fruit and vegetables.) There are also specific points about drinking coffee that are worth mentioning:

★ Caffeine is a diuretic, causing the kidneys to excrete more fluid than normal, and so a regular heavy intake can cause significant dehydration over time. For the same reason caffeine is not a good way to replace fluid after exercise.

★ Coffee and tea can interfere with the absorption of iron into the body. If you are prone to anaemia and drink either of these, always try to do so at least an hour before eating rather than an hour afterwards.

★ Pregnant women should avoid caffeine if possible as it crosses the placenta and enters the baby, as well as being transferred into breast milk.

★ Suddenly stopping drinking coffee can cause caffeine withdrawal, which is marked by symptoms such as headache, fatigue, tiredness and nausea. However, the problem is resolved by gradually cutting down on the number of cups drunk rather than quitting all at once.

★ The key is moderation. My advice to patients is not necessarily to stop drinking coffee but to keep their consumption to no more than two or three cups a day and always use quality brewed coffee rather than instant or heavily processed blends. In this way it is possible to enjoy the mildly stimulating effect without worrying about health issues.

Coffee probably does little harm in moderation. However, if it is part of a lifestyle that also includes smoking, little exercise and a poor diet, you should lose the habit early, before concentrating on the rest.

Get your calcium

I am sure that I say 'Drink your milk' to my children far less often than my parents said it to me, but the principle remains a good one. The main benefit of milk is its calcium content, and although drinking pints of full-fat milk is not a good idea, what is clear is that calcium is crucial in building – and keeping – a healthy skeleton. Although the prevention of osteoporosis is one of the best-known reasons for keeping calcium levels high, it is often forgotten that calcium itself is crucial for the smooth functioning of our muscles, heart and nerves, as well as for healthy teeth.

It is also not realised that nearly 99% of our body's calcium is contained in our bones, and without a steady intake of dietary calcium our bones begin to use up this supply, which causes bone thinning if allowed to continue. A lack of dietary calcium often begins in young girls during dieting fads, and this is a crucial time for bones to reach their maximum weight and density. After the age of 30, bone mass slowly starts to fall and this loss can be accelerated in later years when elderly people stop drinking milk or have a reduced appetite and so are prone to nutritional deficiencies. Because the absorption of calcium is connected with vitamin D – necessary for the normal metabolism of calcium in the body – fortified dairy products and sunlight are important. This means that the housebound and those living in dull Northern climates are especially at risk of not having a healthy calcium turnover.

The easiest way to make sure enough calcium is going into your system is to eat dairy products such as milk, yoghurt and cheese, but if you do not like these, or have a high cholesterol level and have been advised to avoid them, you should eat dark-green, leafy vegetables, figs and almonds, which are all rich in calcium. There is also a huge range of foods fortified with calcium specifically aimed at vegetarians. Almost anyone is able to maintain a good intake of dietary calcium by eating permutations of dairy products, fortified foods, fresh fruit, vegetables and nuts. However, for those people who find that, for one reason or another, they are unable to take the calcium they need, over-the-counter calcium supplements are easy to use. These should be taken with meals to aid absorption, but it is always sensible to check with your doctor first if you are taking other medication or have kidney problems.

Calcium is crucial not only for strong bones but also for the efficient functioning of our muscles, heart and nerves. Make sure your diet contains calcium-rich elements, and take a supplement if your intake of calcium is poor.

Why do they call it the F-Plan Diet, Doctor?

I expect everyone remembers the craze for the F-Plan Diet back in the 1980s, when we were all supposed to eat nothing but fibre and feel wonderful. Since this diet can be somewhat anti-social in its early stages, it was not altogether enthusiastically received in all quarters. Nevertheless, its basic principle remains unchanged today – fibre is good for you. A diet rich in fibre may reduce your risk of developing bowel cancer by up to 40%, according to the biggest study ever undertaken on diet and cancer. The EPIC study, which looked at 400,000 people in nine European countries, studied eating habits and measured consumption of fibre of any type. Those people found to be at the lowest risk of cancer ate half as much fibre again as the average, with 470 people out of the total developing cancer of either the colon or the rectum since they joined the study. These findings back up what has long been thought, but which fell out of favour somewhat several years ago: that fibre is an integral part of a healthy diet.

For this reason we should all aim not only to eat at least five portions of fresh fruit and vegetables each day, but also to include wholegrain bread and cereals in our daily intake. There can be a temporary increase in abdominal distension, flatulence and diarrhoea if the amount of fibre in the diet is increased too quickly, especially if someone is not used to eating it, but these are temporary effects and usually wear off as the body adjusts. It is also important to remember that fibre without fluid equals concrete, and so to prevent constipation it is vital to drink a good quantity of water along with your food. Eight large glasses (eight fluid ounces) a day is the recommended amount.

Current thinking confirms what I have always believed about

sensible eating and diets. Rather than slavishly following certain diets that concentrate on one particular aspect (such as low fat, low carbohydrate, low protein and so on), our bodies are designed to function best on a well-balanced diet in which everything is eaten in moderation and is as fresh as possible. Simple, really.

Be sure to eat fibre regularly. This is essential to a well-balanced diet and can dramatically reduce your risk of bowel cancer.

Oily fish

What do the Inuit people of Greenland and Italians have in common? Absolutely no idea? I didn't know the answer either until I came to write this tip, so we're in good company. Well, let me put you out of your misery and say that it's oily fish. Basically, eating this type of fish appears to reduce the risk of sudden death among heart patients by up to half, which is certainly not a statistic to be sneezed at. Italian researchers looked at the effect of eating omega-3 fatty acids on more than 11,000 heart-attack sufferers. These fatty acids are found in oily fish such as mackerel, salmon and tuna and have long been thought to be beneficial to health and circulation. The results of the study were striking in that the doctors found that a daily dose of one gram of omega-3 fatty acids was enough to reduce the risk of sudden death from a heart attack by over 40%. This appeared to be due to a reduction in irregular heartbeats caused by problems with a pacemaker in the first few months after a heart attack. It was in this crucial early period that the most benefit was noted, and by the end of the three-year study the risk of sudden death was 2% for those people who took fish-oil supplements but 2.7% for those who did not. Every participant in the study ate a sensible Mediterranean-type diet, rich in olive oil, fish and fresh fruit and vegetables, but the addition of fish oil seemed to make a significant difference despite this.

Why should oily fish protect the heart? Although hard fact is still relatively scarce, the current best guess is that omega-3 fatty acids help to regulate the electrical activity in heart cells. An imbalance between different types of fatty acids may cause a tendency to heart irregularities, although the jury is still out on this.

So where do the Greenland Inuit come into all this? Well, back in the 1970s it was recognised that they were doing something right as far as their health was concerned. For it was found that they suffered less from significant illnesses such as heart disease, diabetes and arthritis than their counterparts in the rest of Europe. When their diet was analysed it became clear that they ate large amounts of high-fat food such as whale and seal, which should in theory have increased their risk of illness, but these foods are all rich in omega-3 fatty acids and these had a protective effect on their bodies.

Some doctors have gone as far as to say that eating oily fish is better than using drugs on heart patients. I would not go to such extremes, but there is no doubt that this simple addition to your diet can greatly improve your well-being. Try it and see.

Oily fish contain omega-3 fatty acids, which appear to be crucial in helping to reduce the risk of heart disease. Good examples are tuna, salmon and mackerel.

Always remember the fats of life

If there is one thing I am asked about more than any other when discussing diet or weight-reduction programmes for my patients it is cholesterol. And yet close questioning reveals that most people actually have little knowledge about cholesterol in its various forms apart from the fact that too much is bad for you. This is true enough, but a recent study conducted in Tokyo has shown that the secret of living to be 100 could be more closely linked to cholesterol than we had previously realised. In this study the blood cholesterol levels of 75 centenarians were measured and compared with those of a group 40 years younger. Not only were the general levels of cholesterol lower in the 100-year-olds, but their balance of 'good' and 'bad' cholesterol was better too.

Ah, yes – good and bad cholesterol. This is where it starts to get confusing for many patients (and indeed some doctors). 'Good' cholesterol is more correctly known as HDL or high-density lipoprotein, whereas 'bad' cholesterol is called LDL or low-density lipoprotein. The difference between these two is that good old HDL is said to bind together with another lipoprotein in the body to carry cholesterol away from the tissues and into the liver, which destroys it. The 'bad' LDL does the reverse, pushing cholesterol out into the body tissues and the circulation.

But what does this mean in practice and, more importantly, why did Japanese doctors jump up and down with excitement when they read the results of the study? Well, diet now appears to play a major role in the levels of both good and bad cholesterol *despite* any genetic tendency to have one type of cholesterol present in greater quantity than the other. Looking at what the centenarians ate showed why. Their diet was much richer in foods such as oily fish, porridge, beans and lentils, which help to reduce LDL levels, than that of the younger group. However, it also seems that not only were they lowering their bad cholesterol but also actively pushing up their good cholesterol levels without real-ising it. Their low but steady consumption of nuts – especially almonds – as well as olive oil and avocados, meant that they were taking in regular mono-unsaturated fatty acids, which help to raise HDL levels.

It is not surprising to learn that such foods are chemically sim-ilar to red wine in this regard, acting as antioxidants on the blood. This reduces the amount of LDL being oxidised and turned into plaque on the walls of our arteries, and furred-up pipes equals heart disease, which kills a third of the UK's population every year. So although it is only part of the heart-disease jigsaw, those Tokyo centenarians were doing something different from us, and I can sum it up in one word. Nuts.

Eating foods that increase and maintain LDL, or 'good' cholesterol, is a major way of promoting healthy living. Wash your regular and moderate intake of olive oil, almonds, oily fish, nuts and avocados down with a glass of red wine and your body will thank you for it.

Perspective and diet

I believe that one of the most healthy things any of us can do in our lives is to have a sense of perspective. Whether this is mental, physical or dietary does not matter – the trouble is that all too often we focus on the tiny things while ignoring the big picture, and healthy eating is no exception. Thousands of people spend time, money and effort searching for the perfect diet when in fact no such thing exists and what is needed is a clear idea of what should be eaten more often than not. The simple way of eating, based on seasonal fruit and vegetables allied to wholegrains, pulses and the correct type of fats, works for most people and, with this in mind, I give you the Henderson Perspective Diet, or the A–J Diet:

★ Add salt to food at your peril. This is a powerful cause of high blood pressure and most Western foods contain too much. Keep the salt cellar off the table and avoid adding salt if possible.

★ Breakfast is a vital meal. Porridge, yoghurt or wholegrain toast will set your body up for the day.

★ Cut down on the number of processed and ready-made foods you eat, and increase the proportion of freshly prepared meals.

★ Drink at least eight large glasses (eight fluid ounces) of water each day to help to flush away body toxins. The body is mostly water and in fact needs this more than food.

★ Eat at least five servings of fresh fruit and vegetables each day. I'm not talking about a whole pineapple here. A broccoli spear or a small apple counts as a serving.

★ Fish should be eaten three times a week if possible, preferably of the oily type such as mackerel.

★ Go steady on the amount of alcohol you drink. Aim for a maximum of 21 units per week for men and 14 units per week for women. One unit is equivalent to a single measure of spirit, half a pint of beer or a standard glass of wine.

★ Have no more than six cups of tea, coffee or caffeinated soft drinks each day.

★ In most weeks, eat red meat sparingly – try to have two to three portions a week only.

★ Just replace butter and animal fats in your diet whenever you can with vegetable oils and virgin olive oil.

Never skip meals if at all possible, as this simply makes the body think it is being starved and does you no good at all. Regular meals help to regulate digestion and sleep. Remember that your body is a machine. A complex and wonderful one, to be sure, but still a machine, and like any machine it needs to be looked after properly and have the proper fuel put into it to function properly and for a long time.

Don't slavishly follow diets. Instead, set up healthy eating patterns that then become second nature to you. Your body will love you for it and keep going longer.

Vitamins R, D and A

I recently had a patient who asked me whether she needed vitamins R, D and A. Feeling somewhat uneasy – had I missed the exciting new discovery of vitamin R? – I enquired further and she told me that she had read about the need for a vitamin RDA. Collapse into laughter of doctor and patient followed once this was explained to her.

RDA stands for recommended daily allowance, and refers to the minimum amount of a given vitamin an 'average' adult should need each day to avoid a vitamin deficiency. The vitamin industry believes you need many times the quoted RDA to achieve peak health and so supplements are often set at a much higher dose. Regardless of any hard scientific facts, we in the West are turning into health-supplement junkies, with the UK alone spending at least £360 million on them every year – a rise of over £100 million from five years ago.

We all need vitamins since they are absolutely essential for the normal functioning of our body cells and we are unable to manufacture any ourselves. (The notable exception here is vitamin D, which is manufactured when we sunbathe.) Our bodies therefore depend on us providing enough vitamins in our diet to keep us healthy and, if we do not, there are many possible consequences, ranging from scurvy to rickets and worse. The obvious question here is, if we are eating a sensible diet rich in fresh fruit and vegetables, do not smoke and are exercising regularly, should we need vitamin supplements at all? The answer is probably not, but this does not stop most people from taking them. For this reason it is worth listing some points to bear in mind if you are already taking vitamins or thinking about starting:

★ It probably makes a difference when vitamins are taken. As a general rule it is best to take them first thing in the morning with breakfast. If this is not possible, try to take them with, or close to, another meal.

★ Taking vitamins with a meal is essential in the case of vitamins A, D and E, because these are fat-soluble and so need fat from food to assist their breaking down and digestion. With vitamin C, a light meal is better than a heavy one.

★ Taking the occasional supplement when you remember simply will not work. To gain any benefit at all you need to take vitamins regularly for at least three months.

★ The B group of vitamins have certain peculiarities in that their effects are all counteracted by alcohol, stress and antibiotics. Also, you should not take individual B vitamins unless you are also using a general vitamin B complex. For supplements as a whole, caffeine and smoking usually render any benefits useless, so do not think that you will be able to put right an unhealthy lifestyle by taking a few vitamin tablets.

★ Always be wary of taking too many individual minerals such as zinc or copper. Use a multi-mineral supplement instead. This will reduce the risk of toxic effects from an excess of certain minerals. Remember that vitamins and minerals are different things. Minerals, among which are calcium, iron and zinc, help vitamins to work.

★ If you are pregnant, do not take any supplements without consulting your doctor. The exception is folic acid, which is recommended to be started before conception.

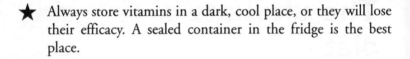

★ Always store vitamins in a dark, cool place, or they will lose their efficacy. A sealed container in the fridge is the best place.

This is one of those areas of health where you pay your money, literally, and you take your choice. Nevertheless, you should be aware that supplements are no match for a well-balanced diet and regular exercise. But if you feel they benefit you, stick to the approved doses, avoid taking cocktails of tablets and read about the properties, benefits and drawbacks of any supplement before starting to take it.

The ultimate anti-ageing diet

Whenever I am engaged in one of my favourite pastimes, browsing in bookshops, I am always amazed at the number of shelves groaning under the weight of diet books. As far as I can make out, these certainly help people to lose pounds, but unfortunately it's usually from their wallets rather than their waistline. I idly wondered about writing the ultimate diet book and got very excited when I thought I was on to something here, but I was beaten to it by decades by people living on the Japanese island of Okinawa. Here there are more centenarians than in any other part of the world, and a population with the world's longest life expectancy – around 85. What is more, most of these elderly people are fitter than their younger Western counterparts.

Equally impressive are the island's health statistics. The population has five times less heart disease than the West and almost half the rate of cancer, as well as cholesterol levels that are some of the lowest in the world. The men have a third more of the male hormone testosterone at the age of 70 than Americans of the same age, and enjoy all the benefits of such levels.

So what is the secret? Well, there is no magic potion or anti-ageing brew that is doing the trick here but rather a simple lifestyle that includes a near-perfect diet and mental approach to life. At first glance the diet appears odd, with a high consumption of foods such as bitter melon and turmeric tea, but it is actually a fusion of Eastern and Western diets that can be readily summarised.

First of all, the Okinawans' calorie intake is 30% less than ours in the West. Not surprisingly, this reduces obesity to almost zero

69

and promotes lean body mass. Secondly, they eat an average of seven servings of fruit and vegetables a day, along with a high quantity of grains and oily fish. Thirdly, there is minimal intake of meat and dairy products, along with a tiny amount of salt – less than three teaspoons per day. Key foods include garlic, ginger, onions, tomato, fish and soya beans – a classic example of a diet rich in flavonoids and antioxidants. It is these substances that appear to be so effective in cutting heart disease and cancer, and which our diet so often lacks.

However, diet alone would not account for such longevity. Allied to this is a moderate but consistent programme of exercise, with a heavy emphasis on martial arts, meditation and stress-relieving exercises such as stretching and deep breathing. There is also a strong social network, which brings all the benefits of being able to talk, laugh and cry with good friends.

Now, we are hardly all going to rush off to the local supermarket to stock up on funny-tasting teas and t'ai chi videos, but there are important principles here for any of us who want to live longer while remaining fit, active and well. One of these is that the typical Western diet is geared to harming our bodies rather than helping them. Another is that one thing alone is not a panacea for a healthy life. A healthy body depends as much on the mind, on taking responsibility for one's own health and on strong community support as anything else, and you won't get too much of these on a prescription. The secret seems to be out there. We have to choose if we want to do anything about it.

If a whole population seems to live longer than any other group of people in the world, it makes sense to sit up and take notice. There's nothing mysterious about the Okinawans' lifestyle – just a common-sense diet allied to a positive mental outlook and exercise. Why didn't we think of it?

More tea, Vicar?

It is time to confess – I am an addict. No less a person than Dr Samuel Johnson predicted my situation when he talked of the 'hardened and shameless tea-drinker, who has for years diluted his meals with only the infusion of this fascinating plant: whose kettle has scarcely time to cool: who with tea amuses the evening, with tea solaces the midnight, and with tea welcomes the morning'. I can think of few things more quintessentially British than a good old-fashioned cup of tea, but our favourite tipple may be better for us than we think, helping to stave off heart disease, cataracts and even bowel cancer. However, despite the perception that we all consume gallons of tea each day, we drink only about three and a half cups, whereas current research suggests that drinking four to six cups daily may help to reduce the risk of chronic diseases such as heart disease.

A Scandinavian study showed that, among men between the ages of 50 and 69, drinking four or five cups of tea a day reduced their risk of stroke by 69%. The most recent study, carried out in America, found that the risk of heart attack in people who drank one or more cups of tea a day was half that of those who didn't drink it at all. The apparent reason is that tea – both green and black – is rich in antioxidants, compounds that help the body to fight harmful free radical molecules. An excess of these has been associated with an increased risk of coronary heart disease and some cancers. Tea is very rich in one group of antioxidants called flavonoids, many of which are released into the drink within the first minute of brewing. Drinking three cups of tea daily for a fortnight appears to raise the concentration of flavonoids in the blood by a quarter.

Contrary to popular belief, tea contains significantly less caffeine than coffee, a cup having an average of 40 milligrams of caffeine, compared with 150 in filter coffee and 64 in instant coffee. More than a dozen cups of tea each day is probably an excessive intake of caffeine, although caffeine does not accumulate in the body. Also interesting is a very recent study published in the *Journal of the American Medical Association* which found that the risk of Parkinson's disease appeared to decline consistently with increasing consumption of tea and other caffeine-containing beverages. There is still a great deal to learn about our national institution, but in the meantime it is encouraging to know that we may be doing ourselves a world of good as we sit and sip our cuppa.

The antioxidants found in tea may be partly responsible for reducing the risks of developing major diseases such as bowel cancer and heart disease. Four to six cups a day is a sensible amount, but because tea is a diuretic this should be supplemented with water or juices to keep fluid intake at a healthy level.

Red meat? Just a little

A friend of mine once had lunch at possibly the finest restaurant in Paris. After ordering a medium steak he sat back to enjoy the gastronomic feast about to come his way while ruminating on a particularly fine French claret with his companion. A little later he was nonplussed to find his steak was so rare that it had only just stopped moving, and sent it back to the chef with his compliments. This scenario was repeated another two times while the chef – who seemed to be allergic to switching his oven on – became increasingly irate. Finally, having taken as much as his pride could stand, the chef stormed out of his kitchen to grandly announce, 'You will never enter my restaurant again until you learn to respect the meat!' Exit all parties and, as my friend later said to me, 'I don't mind respecting meat but I don't want to marry it.'

This pleasing story serves to lead me into the subject of red meat in general, and why we should try to avoid eating it every day and with every meal. As a medical student based near a well-known meat market, I became quite used to seeing very large porters eating half a cow three times a day, but this is perhaps not the most balanced diet in the world. The reason is that there is increasing evidence that the consumption of large quantities of red meat over many years may be linked to the development of certain cancers, most notably cancer of the colon or large bowel. Harvard researchers who studied nearly 90,000 women found that those who ate red meat every day were nearly two and a half times more likely to develop colon cancer than those who ate it infrequently. Why this should be so remains an enigma, but the charring of meat may be important here in that potential carcinogens are produced when meat is cooked. High-temperature cooking can cause the release of substances called heterocyclic amines, which are toxic in animals. Not only is there a link to bowel cancer here, but many studies now suggest that a high-meat, high-fat diet could be linked to prostate cancer, although the question of whether it is the fat content or the meat that is implicated is still under analysis.

What to do then? Vegetarianism is one option, but if, like me, you enjoy the taste of meat, it may be prudent to restrict your intake of red meat to three or four ounces a day. It is also wise to consider the way the meat is cooked, reducing your consumption of meat that is cured, smoked or grilled over a direct flame. I still need my Sunday roast, but I am happy to limit my consumption of other red meats during the week.

Meat is rich in protein and minerals, but too much red meat may be bad for you. Try to keep consumption to sensible levels and to avoid eating it every day.

Never forget breakfast

Often I sit down at my surgery desk at the start of my day and without even looking at my patient list I know exactly how I am going to be feeling by the end of the morning. The explanation is very simple – breakfast. I am one of those individuals who seem to be something of a nice cuddly teddy bear when I have breakfast inside me, and a man-eating grizzly when I have missed it for some reason. Fortunately for me, I know there is nothing strange in this, since the old adage 'Eat breakfast like a king, lunch like a lord and supper like a pauper' has a little bit of science in it.

Research suggests that a decent breakfast – such as porridge, wholegrain toast or a low-fat and high-carbohydrate combination – is good for our health in many ways. Eating a hearty breakfast that contains more than a quarter of our daily calories appears to allow us to eat less fat and more carbohydrates during the day than people who skimp on food in the morning. Studies have shown that breakfast eaters also have a higher intake of essential vitamins and minerals, along with lower levels of harmful serum cholesterol. And on the issue of stress, a study of volunteers reported in the *International Journal of Food Science and Nutrition* found that people who consumed cereal for breakfast every day reported feeling better both physically *and* mentally than those who rarely poured themselves a bowl in the morning. Finally, and crucially, bearing in mind that I am trying to help you to live longer, researchers recently reported that people who reach the ripe old age of 100 tend to consume breakfast more regularly than those who skip the first meal of the day.

What makes breakfast so important? There are four important points to remember here:

★ Including fruit in your breakfast increases your chances of reaching the recommended minimum of five servings of fruits and vegetables a day.

★ A bowl of what you fancy does you good. Breakfast cereal is fortified with many vitamins and minerals, including folic acid, which helps to prevent birth defects and which has been linked to lower risk of heart disease and colon cancer.

★ The best breakfast cereals are rich in fibre, and most of us eat too little of this, despite its obvious long-term health benefits.

★ Breakfast helps us to stay trim. Sitting down to a healthy, high-fibre breakfast is good for the waistline. High-fibre foods fill you up on fewer calories, as well as slowing the digestive process, which in turn wards off hunger pangs later in the morning. In a recent study volunteers were asked to begin their day with a bowl of either cornflakes (which are relatively low in fibre) or oatmeal (which is rich in fibre). Three hours later both groups were invited to take a snack. Those who had had oatmeal for breakfast consumed nearly half of what the other group took.

If you are wondering which kind of breakfast is best, just make sure it includes at least one, but preferably two, servings of fruit, along with high-fibre foods such as granary bread, high-fibre breakfast cereal, or porridge.

Never forget the importance of eating a good breakfast. This helps to reduce stress and the temptation to snack later, and a high-fibre, low-fat breakfast has long-term health benefits.

The Mediterranean diet

A topic that is of interest to many of my patients is the effect of the food they eat on their well-being, and I am asked specific questions about diet two to three times each day in my surgery. Recent research suggests that diet may be even more important in preventing strokes and circulatory problems than was previously thought. Two important points emerge from this work. The first is that three servings a day of wholegrain, such as pasta, cereal or wholegrain bread, almost halve the risk of stroke. Secondly, high quantities of vitamins and antioxidants such as those found in fresh fruit and vegetables should be our dietary aim, so as to help the body to function to its best ability. This area of health has been further highlighted by recent reports that antioxidants in the form of blueberries appear to slow the ageing process in rats.

In a nutshell, normal biological processes linked to the transport of oxygen can form molecules in our cells called free radicals. These have been implicated in a number of diseases, including heart disease, cancer and dementia, but are usually controlled by antioxidants that protect the body from them. These antioxidants are found in vitamins A, C and E, red wine and some plants, and this is probably the reason for the beneficial nature of the so-called 'Mediterranean diet', with its abundance of fruit, vegetables, olive oil and garlic and a healthy amount of wine. This traditional diet is well known to be associated with a reduced risk of heart disease, obesity, gallstones, certain cancers and diabetes. There is considerable debate about the effectiveness of adding vitamin supplements to the diet. My view is that these do little harm, but it is better to try to obtain minerals and vitamins through diet whenever possible. Unfortunately for many people in the West, the main components of their diet are appalling, either through cost, necessity or convenience. In the UK, for example, we eat a diet rich in fat, salt and processed foods and suffer the subsequent health problems that arise from it, including colorectal and breast cancers. The proteins and fats we consume tend to be from animals, whereas in the Mediterranean diet a high proportion of both of these is derived from vegetables.

Many books have been written on the 'perfect' diet, but there are simple ways to both increase the amount of antioxidants we eat and reduce our risks of heart disease, obesity, dementia and possibly some cancerous changes in cells.

We should all aim to eat at least five portions of fresh fruit and vegetables each day, and oily fish twice a week. Do not restrict yourself to one or two favourite foods but aim for variety in your diet, eating pasta, wholegrain bread, potatoes, rice and nuts. Reducing the amount of saturated fat in your diet is important, so choose lean meat and poultry as well as lower-fat dairy foods. Keeping salt off the dining table is sensible, as is drinking alcohol regularly but in moderation. This is simply a sensible eating plan that has the bonus of being high in antioxidants and is therefore beneficial to the body. The dictum 'Man is what he eats' is as valid today as it was when it was first said 150 years ago.

The 'Mediterranean diet' is not a specific regime. It is simply a healthy pattern of eating, based on fresh fruit and vegetables, olive oil, grains and pulses, that helps the body to function at its optimum level. Try it – and don't forget the red wine!

Ignore the salt cellar and the salt sellers

I have been fortunate enough to have eaten in some of the finest restaurants. But while I am always determined to enjoy such experiences to the maximum (especially as I have the ghost of my bank manager standing next to me, wincing at my every mouthful), I am occasionally stopped in my tracks by an occurrence so commonplace that it may seem odd to mention it here. This is the sight of fellow diners lavishly pouring salt all over their food before they have even tasted it. They might as well have stayed at home and poured salt on to any food they chose to and saved themselves the time and expense of going out, since salt actually destroys subtle flavours as effectively as garlic. If someone has more money than sense or taste buds, good luck to them.

What concerns me much more is the fact that 80% of our salt intake is hidden in processed foods and so is unavoidable for many people. It is almost impossible to believe that the food industry will stop adding unnecessarily large amounts of salt to staple foods such as cereals, bread and convenience or ready-made meals despite the well-recognised harmful effects of salt, including high blood pressure (now affecting 15% of the world's population), osteoporosis in women, kidney disease, fluid retention and heart failure. Bearing in mind that we all have to eat and that for most of us a personal low-salt chef is not presiding over our kitchen, what can we do to reduce our risk and so increase longevity?

The first and most obvious thing to do is to remove the salt cellar from the table. This will cut down, on average, around 10% of daily salt intake and is a simple habit to drop. (This truth was demonstrated by an Australian study in a canteen where the hole in the salt cellars was reduced in size. Accordingly, the usual unthinking number of shakes delivered only half the normal quantity of salt. And guess what – nobody noticed the difference.)

Secondly, stop adding salt when cooking. This may be a little harder to achieve since it usually involves breaking a culinary habit of a lifetime. At first, food may taste bland, but most people report a heightened sensitivity to salt after a few weeks, to the extent that it begins to taste most unpleasant. The pattern will be familiar to people who have given up putting sugar in their tea or coffee.

The final, and by far the most difficult step, is to buy as few salt-rich processed foods as possible, including children's foodstuffs. This involves buying as much fresh food as possible and reading the labels on foods more closely. Aim to eat a maximum of six grams of salt a day, and less if possible. For those of us who lead busy lives, this is not easy, but any reduction is beneficial. And so we come back once more to my faithful old medical maxim – moderation is all. Next time you spill the salt, chuck the whole cellar over your shoulder!

Keep your salt intake to a minimum. Salt raises your blood pressure and predisposes you to other chronic medical problems.

Me? Eat chocolate?

I like chocolate. No, let me rephrase that. I am a fully paid-up chocoholic who feels deprived if a day goes by without this wonderful and versatile substance passing my lips. Apart from being the only food that melts at body temperature, it may also – and this is almost too good to be true – help you to live longer.

I know what you're thinking. How on earth can a calorie-soaked, fat-rich, chocolate fudge possibly be good for me? Well, that's the point – it isn't. I'm not talking here about the typical chocolate bar or chocolate-based confectionery found in every newsagent and supermarket in the land. If you are going to get any benefit from chocolate, there are, unfortunately, two basic rules to observe. The first is to eat only small quantities. The second is to eat the finest-quality chocolate you can afford, with a cocoa content of at least 60%. This has less saturated fat than the typical milk chocolate preferred in the UK and so has a more bitter taste than many people are used to.

It has been known for many years that there is a link between, on the one hand, antioxidants in chocolate, and, on the other hand, a reduction in blood 'stickiness' and an increase in levels of 'good' cholesterol. The thinking is that eating the right kind of chocolate can actually reduce the risk of heart disease. In the past year, scientific trials unveiled at the world's largest general science meeting suggest that chocolate may also help to reduce high blood pressure. The evidence comes from a group of Kuna Indians living off the coast of Panama, who drink large quantities of a particularly raw and unprocessed type of cocoa. This is similar to high-quality dark, bitter chocolate, which is packed with flavonols – a sub-group of the naturally occurring substances known as flavonoids. Flavonols appear to be able to affect levels of nitric oxide in the body, which in turn is vital for the maintenance of healthy blood pressure and cardiovascular health. So, cocoa with a high flavonol content – from which dark chocolate is made – is thought to help to dilate blood vessels and so reduce blood pressure.

Before the blood pressure of any doctor reading this goes through the roof, I give this caveat – as with so many things that are good for you, moderation is all. This is no excuse to pig out on left-over selection boxes and an extra bar or two of your favourite chocolate each day. Rather, it is an invitation to eat a few pieces of high-quality dark chocolate every day and enjoy them without worry.

I should have remembered this fact when I bumped into an obese patient of mine outside a corner shop. She was happily unwrapping a large bar of chocolate, but when I raised my eyebrows at her she had the grace to look rather guilty, doubtless recalling the long consultations she had had with me about her inability to lose weight. But before I could say anything, she simply said, 'It's all right, Doctor, I only eat it slowly, so less calories go in', then trundled off to enjoy her feast. I still don't know whether to laugh or cry.

Chocolate may be an indulgence, but a little of what you fancy – provided it's of high quality – may actually do you some good.

Spice up your life

I ate very few 'foreign' foods when I was young, and the first time I went to London as a teenager and ate a pizza I thought it was the height of exotic gastronomy. Fortunately, my palate has broadened since then to include what people have been eating for thousands of years – spices. Ethnobotanists, who look at the health-giving properties of plants, believe that certain spices not only make food taste better but can also improve your health and well-being. This is mainly because of their anti-bacterial and anti-microbial properties, which are especially useful in hot countries, but there are also deeper benefits. A great many spices offer benefits for health, but a small number of them I believe to be particularly beneficial, although this is only my personal view.

The best 'all-round' anti-bacterials are probably oregano, onion, allspice and garlic, as they kill the vast majority of micro-organisms found on meat. Thyme, cinnamon and tarragon are also effective here to some degree, as are chillies and peppers.

Garlic really is a valuable spice, as it contains allicin, a potentially powerful anti-cancer agent. In addition it has been implicated in lowering blood pressure and helping to reduce cholesterol. Not surprisingly, it also seems to prevent the transmission of glandular fever – sometimes called 'the kissing disease'!

Cumin contains the anti-cancer agents carevol and limonene, which may give protection against prostate cancer, and sage is also rich in beneficial antioxidants as well as being used to treat coughs and colds. Parsley contains significant amounts of histadine, which is said to inhibit tumours and also helps to reduce blood pressure and increase urine production.

Red peppers contain capsaicin – a hugely beneficial chemical in the treatment of arthritis and pain in general, so much so that an extract of this is now available on prescription in the

UK. Turmeric is similarly useful, as well as having strong anti-inflammatory properties. Thyme is available in extract form in various cough and cold remedies as thymol oil, which has been used as a germicide since the early twentieth century.

Ginger has long been recommended to me by patients as a very helpful treatment for travel sickness, but it also contains the antioxidants gingerol and zingerone. The latter is said to react with free radicals to help to prevent the damage that these can cause to tissue cells.

The list is long and varied, but the basic premise is the same – spices are better for you than you may realise. We in the West often take the view that a hot curry is the way to eat spices, but my Indian colleagues eat them in a much more subtle, milder and healthier way, and I prefer to follow their example.

Spices have more health benefits than we realise. We do not need to eat them with every meal, but, taken little and often, they are good for us.

Try the DASH diet

From behind my desk I hear about all types of diet – weird, wonderful and downright dangerous. There are occasions when people seem to have a need to stick slavishly to some particular diet rather than be able to do all that dieting requires – to eat less. However, for those of you who prefer to lose weight by following a 'plan', let me gently steer you towards a type of diet which most people find simple and easy, and which did not raise my blood pressure too much when I first heard about it. Like many diets, it comes from America, and it was christened the DASH diet after the Dietary Approaches to Stop Hypertension study carried out there. Putting it at its simplest, this is a diet low in saturated fats and rich in fruits, vegetables and low-fat dairy products. As a result of this combination, it is low in cholesterol, high in fibre and moderately high in protein, and has good levels of potassium, magnesium and calcium. Although it was originally aimed at people with high blood pressure or heart disease, there is, unusually, enough common sense in this diet for me to be happy to recommend it generally.

For calorie counters among you, it adds up to approximately 2,000 calories per day. It should include most of the following:

★ Five servings of fresh fruit each day.

★ Seven servings of grains each day.

★ Five servings of fresh vegetables each day.

★ Two servings of lean meat, poultry and fish each day.

★ Two or three servings of low-fat dairy products each day.

★ Five servings of nuts, legumes and seeds each week.

★ Very limited amounts of sweets and saturated fats.

You don't need a science degree to understand that. But what is scientific is that one study showed that eight weeks of this diet lowered users' systolic blood pressure by an average of 11 millilitres Hg and diastolic blood pressure by an average of five millilitres Hg – a reduction that many doctors would find acceptable when treating patients with anti-hypertensive drugs. A combination of antioxidants (fresh fruit and vegetables) and a component for healthy circulation (low-fat, high grain) seems to do the trick, as well as being reasonably low in calories. Don't make it too complicated, though – we are simply machines and food is our petrol. We simply need to make sure that we are using the best fuel we can.

If you desperately need a diet plan to hold on to in order to lose weight, try the DASH diet. As well as promoting weight loss, it helps to reduce blood pressure, which in many people is one of the key factors in early death from heart disease.

Eat mood food

When I was at school I was once asked to write an essay about the premise that we are what we eat. I cannot remember my reply, although I think it was something along the lines of 'If you eat lots of carrots you'll go orange'. However, the old adage is pretty much true, and this applies to our mental health as well as our physical.

Doctors have known for some time that the healthy functioning of our brain, along with associated mood changes, depends on the correct supply of nutrients reaching our brain cells. 'Eat fish for your brains' is a phrase I still hear, and this is true because of the high nutrient content of fish. However, fish does not supply a key nutrient for good mental health – thiamine. A lack of thiamine in the diet is frighteningly common, with half of both young adults and pensioners being short of it to the point of clinical deficiency at any one time, although very often the symptoms are not attributed to this problem. In fact many doctors (including me) do not routinely consider thiamine deficiency as a diagnosis and this situation is not helped by the fact that symptoms are often linked to many other common conditions. Most sufferers report irritability and temper tantrums, weight loss, muscle weakness and depression or long periods of low mood for no obvious reason. One study of thiamine deficiency gave university students a thiamine supplement every day for two months, and, somewhat to their surprise, the investigators found that the students reported significant improvements in mood and energy levels over this time. This could be due partly to a placebo effect, but the results were confirmed in older people when they were given a lower dose of thiamine.

As a general rule, highly processed foods tend to contain very little thiamine, so avoid or cut down on these. To make sure your levels of thiamine do not drop too low, eat plenty of wholegrains and cereals, as well as some meat, such as lean pork. Many people believe they are eating correctly in this way but are undoing all their good work by drinking lots of tea or coffee, which interfere with the body's absorption of thiamine. Drink no more than six cups a day of either, and fewer if you can. A sensible maximum for coffee is less than 350 milligrams of caffeine per day (an average cup of instant coffee contains 60 milligrams of caffeine, and an average cup of filter coffee up to 150 milligrams).

Other good 'mood minerals' include vitamin B12, folic acid, selenium, iron (often very low in many people without their being aware of it) and vitamin C. These may work by improving the production of a brain chemical called serotonin, which is known to be a crucial factor in depression and mood.

With depression and stress becoming ever more common, anything that can be done in a simple way to reduce this risk should be done, and few things are simpler than watching what you eat.

'Mood foods' contain key minerals and supplements that appear to help the brain to produce depression-beating chemicals. It is particularly important to get enough thiamine in your diet and to avoid eating too much highly processed food and drinking too much tea or coffee.

Homo what?

Ask the average person what homocysteine is and you will probably get an enquiring raise of the eyebrows at best. The body makes this chemical waste product during the process of methylation, which is a vital part of cellular function. Stick with me – the science bit is nearly over. In excess, homocysteine can circulate in the bloodstream and dramatically increase the risk of both dementia and heart disease. It is certainly not something you would want building up over the long term, but fortunately there does appear to be a way of helping to reduce its effects on our health. The answer is dietary and relies on the body having enough folic acid and vitamins B6 and B12 – these are all found in fresh fruit and vegetables – to convert it back to something called glusathione, one of the body's good guys. This powerful antioxidant helps the body to remove harmful free radicals caused by smoking, drinking and a generally unhealthy lifestyle.

What simple things can we do with our diet to keep this cellular process on the right track? Well, as scientists continue to find out more about homocysteine and its links to dementia and heart disease, the sensible thing to do is alter your diet to include more dark-green, leafy vegetables, low-fat dairy products, wholegrain bread and citrus fruits. This probably works far better than the random use of supplements, but if you want to use these, make sure you take vitamins B6 and B12 and folic acid.

With dementia (especially Alzheimer's disease) and coronary heart disease now so common in the elderly population, anything that can be done simply and effectively to reduce the risk of these should be encouraged. It is good to know that excess homocysteine is one of those problems where improvement can sometimes be achieved without high technology or medicines.

Dementia and heart disease are increasingly being linked to the build-up of homocysteine in the body. Reduce this by increasing the amount of dark-green, leafy vegetables and wholegrain in your diet.

Eat up your porridge

Porridge is one of life's great comfort foods – what could be better on a cold and dark winter morning? – but if eaten all year round it has significant benefits for the body.

It has long been known that cereal grain is an important component of any healthy diet, and many of the diets I mention in this book have grains and pulses as part of their framework. The major element in grains – and these include porridge oats – that contributes to health is fibre, especially soluble fibre. In the mid-1990s health experts went so far as to say that this soluble fibre – when eaten as part of a diet low in saturated fats and cholesterol – could reduce the risk of coronary heart disease. So why should this be the case?

The key here is that oats are one of the best sources of a soluble fibre called beta glucan. This is especially good at lowering the level of 'bad' cholesterol in our bloodstream, especially the so-called LDL particles that are notorious for clogging up very fine blood vessels around the body, including our coronary arteries. Like all plant foods, oats contain certain phytochemicals and antioxidants that also help to reduce the risk of heart disease, and in many ways these mimic the action of vitamin E as well as working with it. Such compounds may – in certain people – also counteract the circulatory effects of a high-fat meal by maintaining blood flow and preventing blood-vessel constriction, although this effect is somewhat powerless against a relentless onslaught of fatty food.

Another point where porridge scores highly is that oat fibre may also help to control the level of our blood sugar. It is unclear just how much porridge is required to do this, but it does seem that such a cereal may be an extremely sensible food for people with diabetes or problems of insulin resistance as a result of this condition.

Porridge – with skimmed milk but preferably no salt or sugar – should be a staple component of a staple diet, and eaten regularly rather than just in the winter.

Porridge is an excellent source of soluble fibre. It has been implicated in helping to reduce the risk of heart disease, as well as having other health benefits, such as helping to regulate blood sugar levels and to even out the rate at which food is digested. Try it – you might like it.

Go veggie

There are three absolute certainties in life that I am aware of. The first is death – a constant companion in my professional life. The second is taxes. The third is that I will never become a vegetarian. I sometimes recall a story about George Bernard Shaw, who is said to have declined an invitation to a gala testimonial because the menu was exclusively vegetarian. Although a staunch vegetarian himself, he said that the thought of two thousand people all crunching celery at the same time horrified him.

I happily accept the need for an ethical debate about whether we choose to be carnivores or not, but, having been brought up as a 'meat and two veg' man, I genuinely believe our bodies are designed to run best on a combination of meat, fruit, vegetables and pulses. I am not some kind of meat fanatic who believes all vegetarians weave their own yoghurt, and I can in fact see the health benefits of a vegetarian diet. It's not for me, though. Let me tell you why.

A vegetarian diet has long been recognised as conferring a number of health benefits. Various research projects have shown that vegetarians suffer less heart disease, obesity, high blood pressure and bowel disorders such as diverticulitis and diabetes, to list but a few advantages of such a diet. One study in the mid-1980s found that vegetarians made 22% of the visits to hospital outpatient departments compared to non-vegetarians and spent a similarly low proportion of time in hospital. Why should this be the case? Well, a carefully planned vegetarian diet – if followed to the letter – closely matches the recommended daily intake of fresh fruit and vegetables, complex carbohydrates and antioxidants, as well as being high in fibre and low in saturated fats. (One important point here in my meat-eater's defence is that a carnivore's diet can have exactly this combination but our Western high-fat, highly processed diet can make this difficult to achieve unless we constantly and carefully watch our food intake.)

As a general policy, we should all eat less fat – particularly saturated fats – and increase our consumption of complex carbohydrates and fibre while reducing our sugar and salt intake, and a vegetarian diet usually achieves these aims by default. Vegetarians tend to eat up to 25% less fat each day than non-vegetarians, and obviously less saturated fat since animal products are the major sources of this. The usually greater consumption of fresh fruit and vegetables in a vegetarian diet means that there is a high intake of protective antioxidants such as vitamins A, C and E, which are believed to protect against certain cancers and heart disease. So, all these factors contribute to the general healthiness of vegetarianism, but balance is the key here, and that is why I continue to happily eat meat. My meat intake tends to be fish and organic lean white meat as a supplement to the nutrients found in a vegetarian diet. But if, for whatever reason, you would feel happier to exclude meat from your diet altogether, then you will probably be doing yourself some good in comparison with non-vegetarians who eat a *poor* diet – one that is high in fat, low in fibre, and contains a lot of heavily processed food but only a little fresh fruit and vegetables.

To come full circle to George Bernard Shaw, he once found himself sitting next to J.M. Barrie, the author of *Peter Pan*, at a luncheon. Observing the mound of green, leafy vegetables on Shaw's plate, Barrie leaned over and murmured, 'Tell me, George, have you already eaten that or are you going to?' Shaw had the last laugh – he outlived Barrie by many years.

Vegetarianism can confer health benefits compared with a poor non-vegetarian diet. If it is for you, eat well and widely to get the full advantage.

'Men do not quit playing because they grow old; they grow old because they quit playing.'

– Oliver Wendell Holmes

Lifestyle tips

Flossing is good for you

There are two things I think about when I hear the word 'floss'. The first is a rather lovable mutt of that name who is an integral part of my family. The second is that most tedious of chores, but one which seems to send dentists into raptures – flossing your teeth. I find this one of those jobs that I keep reminding myself to do but always seem to be that little bit too busy to perform, instead going into a flossing frenzy a week before my appointment with the dentist. It will come as no surprise that this has no impact on my dental health and merely serves to raise a knowing smile from my dentist as he pokes and prods my teeth and gums. I really should know better, however, not only because I see enough oral disease in my job to keep reminding me but also because there is now increasing evidence that flossing is beneficial for long-term health and may even protect against heart disease.

Researchers have found that people with periodontal disease (problems such as gum infections or gingivitis) are almost twice as likely to suffer from coronary heart disease as those without such gum conditions. Although the exact reason for this is still being evaluated, it would seem that gum disease causes the release of potentially harmful bacteria into the bloodstream. It is thought that these bacteria can trigger or speed up any furring-up of the arteries in the body that may be already occurring and in extreme cases even cause blood clots. Although it is well known that certain medical conditions, such as rheumatic heart disease, require antibiotic cover before any dental work is undertaken, this research perhaps suggests that flossing may be a simple, cheap and effective way to reduce the risk of heart disease.

But how can you tell if you have gum disease? Well, the usual symptom is bleeding gums during or after brushing your teeth.

If your gums are swollen, tender or red, you may well have a problem, or if someone who is close to you has been candid enough to say you have bad breath, this can also be a sign of gum disease. Further down the line, if gum disease is allowed to continue, teeth may become loose or the way they fit together when you bite can feel different from how it has always been.

Regular dental checks are only half the answer here. Remember to floss every day and to check for signs of gum disease. In this way not only could you still have a full set of teeth as a centenarian but your dental hygiene may have helped you to get to such an age.

Simple things sometimes make a big difference. Although it may seem a chore, regular flossing can help your dental and long-term general health.

Give blood

If I have heard one joke from patients about Dracula or blood-suckers when taking a blood sample, I must have heard a hundred. I also understand that this is the lot of blood transfusion doctors and nurses, who must hear the same thing dozens of times a day and yet still manage to raise a dutiful smile as required. I can only assume that this is the case, though, since one of the cardinal sins of my life – and one I am slightly uncomfortable about confessing to – is that I have never yet become a blood donor. This is not through any lack of wanting to. It is just that whenever the mobile transfusion service is in town I always seem to be sitting behind my desk with a room full of patients next door waiting to see me.

However, in the course of researching this book I came across some interesting information about giving blood, and this may yet have me toddling off across the road to donate. By topping up the national blood bank not only will I be helping to save someone else's life, but I may also be helping to save my own.

In men, regular blood donations can help to reduce excess amounts of iron in the blood. Iron acts as an oxidant in the body, but too much of it can be detrimental to health, which in turn means that lowering its level may be beneficial. The reason is that iron molecules are essential for the formation of what are called oxygen radicals in the body and these have been implicated in cardiovascular disease and other age-related diseases. Lowering the iron load reduces the production of oxygen radicals and so can lead to a reduction in ageing processes at a cellular level. Because men are more prone to producing oxygen radicals than women, this process may also explain in part why pre-menopausal women have a lower incidence of hardening of the arteries (atherosclerosis) and suffer approximately half the number of heart attacks that men do at the same age.

I well remember as a junior hospital doctor approaching the foot of the bed of a very elderly, and very poorly, 88-year-old lady from whom I had to take some blood for diagnostic testing purposes. As I was about to gently wake her up, she opened one eye, fixed my syringes and needles with a stern gaze and said, 'That's all I need right now. Another doctor with just a little prick.'

Giving blood is not only good for the soul but also for the body – yours and that of the grateful recipient of your blood too.

Remember HIV

There is a widespread belief that the only way to make sure sexually transmitted diseases, including HIV, do not affect people is either to live a chaste life or never have sex before marriage. But we live in the real world, and, whatever the merits of this argument, simply believing it isn't going to make it happen. So, although safe-sex precautions are not necessary when neither you nor your partner has anything you could transmit to each other, if you choose to have a number of sexual partners – at any age – your health and peace of mind can be enhanced by playing safe.

The single most effective thing you can do to stay healthy while being sexually active is to use latex condoms for intercourse, whether vaginal or anal. All condoms are not made alike; men (and women) should experiment with different brands until they find the one they like best and know how to use them correctly. For a while health experts were recommending that people choose safer-sex products treated with Nonoxynol-9 to protect against HIV transmission, but the latest scientific evidence suggests that this advice should be formally retracted. It should be obvious, although surprisingly often it is not, that a new condom needs to be used for each new partner, and that condoms should not be reused. Also, if you switch from anal to vaginal intercourse, you should put on a new condom to avoid causing vaginal infections.

Where oral sex is concerned, it is clear that herpes can be transmitted from genitals to mouth or mouth to genitals during unprotected sex, but some medical experts consider that the risk is acceptably low outside of the most infectious period. Very rarely, you can pick up a bacterial infection by having oral sex with someone who has a bacterial sexually transmitted disease (typically gonorrhoea), but these can usually be cured with antibiotics once identified. Fortunately, it is clear that the risk of transmitting HIV is massively lower for unprotected oral sex than for unprotected intercourse, and that the risk is much lower for the person being sucked or licked than for the person doing it. For the person sucking or licking, the risk of transmission is lower if their gums, lips, mouth and throat are healthy. For this reason some sex educators recommend that flossing or brushing the teeth be avoided for an hour before giving unprotected oral sex, as these can cause the gums to bleed, which may bring about blood-to-blood transfer, especially if the sexual activity is vigorous.

There are two sexually transmitted diseases for which vaccination is available: hepatitis B and hepatitis A. Hepatitis B can be spread easily through intercourse and, less easily, through oral sex. Hepatitis A is easily spread through oro-anal contact. Getting these two vaccinations, which you can do at the same time, is an excellent idea if you don't always use protective barriers during these activities.

Outside a monogamous relationship, the rules of safe sex apply to everyone, young or old – sexually transmitted diseases, including HIV, are no respecters of age, class or colour. Always practise safe sex if you need to. Don't die of embarrassment.

Know your healthy weight

You probably know how much you weigh, but if you don't, you can just hop on the scales. Simple enough, you might think, but this is only part of the story, for many doctors are now not relying exclusively on a weight obtained in this way. Rather, they – and I – are increasingly tending to work out whether patients are underweight or overweight by calculating a body mass index, or BMI. All nutritionists agree that each of us has a healthy weight range, outside of which we become more prone to conditions such as high blood pressure, diabetes, heart disease, gallstones and joint problems. If we remain within the healthy range, the chances of these occurring fall, and we are able to choose at what weight within those limits we both look and feel best.

BMI is calculated by a fairly simple arithmetical formula, and charts that help you to do this can be found at your doctor's surgery or in the back of dieting magazines. You simply divide your weight in kilograms by your height in metres squared. So, if you weigh 70 kilograms and are 1.63 metres tall, simply multiply 1.63 by itself and then divide 70 by this figure (2.66) to give a reading of 26.3. This is your BMI.

Ideally, a BMI should be between 20 and 25, the second of five weight ranges:

★ BMI under 20 – underweight. You will be encouraged to gain weight.

★ BMI 20 to 25 – normal. Aim to keep within this category and avoid the temptation to put on a few kilograms each year.

★ BMI 25 to 30 – overweight. Weight loss needs to be considered here, but preferably no more than a kilogram per week.

★ BMI 30 to 40 – obese. Your weight is now affecting your health and will cause significant problems in the future.

★ BMI over 40 – seriously obese. Immediate weight loss is needed, often with the help of professionals. Consult your doctor for advice.

As with all templates, there are caveats. These figures obviously do not apply to pregnant women, or to growing children or teenagers (although obesity in children is an increasing trend). Sportsmen and women can appear to be overweight when in fact they are trim and healthy simply because their higher proportion of muscle weighs more than fat.

At the very least, a BMI allows you to see whether you are in a healthy weight range or not, and, if you aren't, reminds you that you need to do something about it. Weight control really is an excellent investment in your long-term health.

Instead of relying strictly on what your bathroom scales tell you about your weight, calculate your body mass index. Your BMI is a more reliable way of showing whether or not your health is likely to suffer in the future as a result of weight-related conditions.

Keep to a healthy weight

Why do we doctors keep banging on about losing weight or keeping to the weight you are, or telling you, 'Just watch what you eat, young man, or you'll get fat'? Well, if there is one thing that may inch us all towards the magic 100 mark more than anything, it is keeping trim and lean. The problem is that to achieve the maximum benefit you would need to practically starve yourself all your life to stay at an artificially low weight. However, we still get the benefit simply from sticking within the normal ranges seen in body-weight graphs in doctors' waiting rooms and diet magazines.

We have known for many years that if you keep rats underfed (i.e. with a healthy diet, just less of it than usual) from the time they are born, they will live a third longer than their fatter counterparts, as well as being healthier during their extended life. Why should a very low food intake do this? There seems to be a link with the body's metabolic rate and its consumption of oxygen. When your body believes that it is being starved, your metabolic rate drops to try to keep your weight at its present level. This reduces the demand for oxygen from your cells, which then causes the production of fewer free radicals – the damaging by-products of your metabolism.

Scientists who firmly believe that this is the way to a long life and act on it are putting their money where their mouth is. They are trying to live by keeping their weight at about two thirds of what is usually regarded as normal, but my view is that a pragmatic approach to life has to start somewhere and I am quite happy with my weight being three thirds of normal, thank you very much.

As part of the reason why the residents of Okinawa stay well for so long, lean body mass and low body weight are important.

For you and me, though, I don't suggest you starve yourself, but I do suggest not letting yourself become overweight.

Your health will benefit if you stay within the normal weight range for your height. You can work out for yourself – see the previous tip – whether you fall into this range already. If you don't, you may need help from your doctor to reach and stay at a healthy weight.

Keep young and beautiful

I am something of a sucker for old black-and-white documentary films, and the ones about medical issues can give fascinating insights into what were then considered to be the best public health messages available. I remember one in particular which exhorted people to gather in groups and vigorously swing large dumbbells around their heads in freezing conditions – this would apparently 'tone up' the body to prepare you for the day ahead. Prepare you for a visit to the doctor, more likely. Exercise then, as now, is hugely beneficial for the body and the good news is you do not need to knock your neighbour's head off with a heavy weight to tone yourself up.

Most people who exercise regularly will tell you that they feel much better than they did before they began to exercise. There is no doubt that this is partly due to the fact that when we exercise the brain produces chemicals called endorphins. These can bring about a feeling of well-being and good health as well as helping us to cope better with stress and strong emotions. The physical benefits of regular exercise are many, but among the most marked are a slower pulse rate, healthier lungs and increased flexibility. Remember these basic points about exercise:

★ It need take only 20–30 minutes of exercise three times a week for your body to feel the benefits. Any activity that raises the heart rate and gets you gently out of breath and warm will achieve this. You do not need to run a marathon – brisk walking, cycling or, my personal favourite recommendation, swimming, are all fine. If you enjoy it, do it.

★ Don't forget yoga. This benefits both mind and body, and the mind relaxes progressively as the body does an increasing amount of muscular work. Some studies have shown that when large muscle groups repeatedly contract and relax, the brain releases specific neurotransmitters to relax the body more and heighten mental alertness.

★ If you are normally surrounded by people at work or home, a big exercise class may be counterproductive and solo exercise may be best for you. But if you work or live alone, a group activity may do you more good. Find out what works for you.

★ Always warm up before exercising and warm down afterwards, to reduce the chances of pulling a muscle.

★ People who exercise regularly tend to eat more nutritious food than those who do not, which in turn helps them to stay even more healthy and well.

So many millions of words have been written about the benefits of exercise that the message sometimes gets lost through repetition. The best advice remains the same, however – keep it simple, keep it enjoyable and keep it up! When I was running in the London Marathon one year I began to suffer somewhat at the 23-mile mark. Concentrating on putting one foot in front of the other, I was surprised (and a little piqued) to see an old man sail past as if out on a morning jog. As I caught him up, I puffed, 'What's the secret?' Smiling, the 78-year-old said, 'I may look old, but in my head I'm younger than you!' A classic response if ever I heard one.

Exercise need not involve hours of sweating in a gym. Even walking is good for you if done regularly. Make exercise part of your routine and the benefits to your health will follow as night follows day.

Another doctor talking about smoking

If there was just one thing in the world I could change to benefit people's health, it would be to stop people smoking. As smoking is the leading cause of premature death and avoidable illness in the UK, I often find myself on the horns of a dilemma with my nicotine-addicted patients. I can explain the risks of smoking to them until I am blue in the face, but if they choose not to stop, even with the help of smoking clinics, that is their decision and they will live with the health consequences. However, we simply cannot continue to ignore the facts; in the UK there are 1,000 hospital admissions every day for smoking-related diseases, absenteeism due to smoking is responsible for the loss of 34 million working days each year, and – my own personal bugbear – passive smoking causes 17,000 hospital admissions in children under five each year. Figures for Australia are no more encouraging, with just under one million hospital bed-occupation days occurring annually as a result of smoking-related illnesses.

I have no moral objection to adults choosing to smoke of their own free will, but I draw the line at small children being hospitalised because of the actions of their smoking parents. In case I am accused of preaching from the high ground as a non-smoker, I would simply point out that I see the effects of smoking at close quarters every day, and it becomes somewhat depressing to attend the funerals of an endless line of patients who die early because of giving up their cigarettes too late.

So what is to be done? It doesn't seem to matter how much the price of cigarettes rises – the problem of nicotine addiction doesn't go away. And it's worth bearing in mind here that the

World Health Organisation considers nicotine to be more addictive than heroin or cocaine. Less than 20% of smokers who make a serious attempt to stop the habit remain cigarette-free after one year. Most smokers continue to smoke not because they want to but because of their addiction to nicotine, and the best results in breaking this have consistently been shown to be a combination of pharmacological therapy and motivational support. Nicotine replacement therapy (NRT) replaces one type of highly refined nicotine delivery system – the cigarette – with another, safer form, such as a patch or chewing gum, and so allows a gradual weaning off the drug. NRT delivers nicotine less effectively than a cigarette, however, since smoking will send it to the brain within ten seconds – faster than if it was injected intravenously. The advent in the UK of NRT on prescription is to be welcomed, along with other non-NRT medications, but the bottom line is this – if you *really* want to stop smoking, don't be afraid to ask for help. Stopping this habit will be the single most beneficial thing you will *ever* do for yourself and your family.

Smoking kills people very effectively. As I say to patients debating whether or not they want to stop, 'What makes you built any differently from all the others who have died before you?'

Carbon monoxide – the silent killer

It is always a tragedy when a life is cut short by a preventable accident. And this is exactly what happens with a type of fatality which peaks towards the end of the year and which kills a reported 50 people annually – although this is probably an under-estimate – in the UK. The cause is carbon-monoxide poisoning. The autumn and winter are notorious for this kind of accident because of the increased use of gas appliances such as boilers and fires. The groups most at risk tend to be students and the elderly, but anyone can succumb.

Carbon monoxide is so dangerous because it binds to the oxygen-carrying part of our blood much more than oxygen does, as well as progressively destroying brain cells and other cell enzymes. This leads to a gradual onset of symptoms, often subtle, the commonest of which are flu-like symptoms, headaches and tiredness, and gastrointestinal upsets such as diarrhoea and vomiting. It is common for several family members or occupants of the same house to be affected. (Nor are pets immune, though I recall a patient's Labrador dog that suddenly refused to enter the room where there was a faulty gas fire.) If symptoms are left undiagnosed the progressive depletion of oxygen in the blood can prove fatal, often as a result of sleeping overnight in a room with a faulty appliance.

It is a sobering thought that over a quarter of a million gas appliances are officially condemned each year in the UK. Some 20% of these – the figure may well be higher – are emitting potentially fatal amounts of carbon monoxide, which means that at least 50,000 people are currently being poisoned without knowing it. Of even more concern is the fact that when many of these sufferers attend either their doctor or a hospital, the diagnosis is not thought of and they are returned to the very atmosphere that is harming them. (I would have diagnosed the patient I mentioned above as having flu had he not mentioned his wary dog.) The majority of people who die from carbon-monoxide poisoning have seen a doctor about their symptoms but have not been tested for this possibility because of a lack of awareness in both doctor and patient. It is now possible to test for carbon monoxide not only with conventional blood tests but also with new breath tests. Wider availability of such tests, allied to a far greater use of simple and cheap domestic carbon-monoxide alarms, is the way forward in permanently reducing the number of deaths caused by this preventable form of poisoning.

Some killers are more silent than others. Carbon monoxide is the stealthiest of all, so be sure to have gas appliances checked every year by a qualified engineer. It may well save your life.

What's a statin?

Many of my patients are extremely concerned about their cholesterol level, often unnecessarily but just as frequently with good reason. I have been known myself to sidle up to my practice nurse and ask her to take a blood sample 'just to check' my level, even though I am apparently hale and hearty. One of the reasons for my curiosity is that in the UK the average cholesterol level hovers around six millimoles per litre, whereas the accepted upper limit should be 5.2 and many of our European colleagues have levels below four. The reason we need to keep a close watch on cholesterol is that the higher the level, the greater the risk of heart attack and stroke.

Although our diet in this country leaves a lot to be desired, it is not the main reason for high cholesterol levels. Improving your diet may reduce your cholesterol count by 10–15% at best, but the fact is that most people with raised levels simply produce too much themselves. It is the body's natural production of cholesterol that is the problem.

So, if you have dieted as hard as you can and are eating all the low-fat foods you should, what is the next step? Salvation arrives in the form of a group of drugs known as statins, which block the production of cholesterol in the liver by at least a third (often more), and they work quickly too. A recent research project known as the HPS (Heart Protection Study), which looked at 20,000 people in just under 70 British hospitals, showed that taking a statin could reduce the chances of having a heart attack or stroke by 30%. Since 10% of the population have cholesterol levels high enough to warrant treatment with statins, that same 10% should be being prescribed them – right? Wrong. In fact only around 1% of the population takes them and there are a number of reasons for this, with cost being a prime factor.

If GPs in the UK were to prescribe statins for every patient who needed them, this one drug would come very close to breaking the financial back of the NHS. It's sad but true. As a result, patients slip through the net, and family doctors don't exactly go out of their way to throw these drugs at you. However, there are groups of people who are at particular risk and I always try to make sure that they have statin cover. If you have a high cholesterol level and think you might be in such a group, discuss the possibility of statin treatment with your doctor. The signs to look out for are:

★ A strong family history of heart attacks below the age of 55.

★ A history of heart attacks or angina.

★ High blood pressure.

★ Diabetes.

★ A family history of high cholesterol levels.

**A high cholesterol level can be dramatically reduced –
along with the risk of heart attack and stroke – by
medication known as statins, but not everyone who needs
these is prescribed them. If you have a high cholesterol
level and do not take them, ask your doctor whether they
should be prescribed for you.**

Genetic testing

Medical care today is so different from 50 years ago that most family doctors from that time would hardly recognise what I do most days in my surgery. But this change will be as nothing compared with what happens over the next half-century, and at the forefront of medical advances will be genetic testing and treatments. However, as far as this book is concerned, there is a caveat here, and that is the question, 'Will genetic testing actually help me to live longer?' The short answer is probably not, although it is obvious that if a serious condition is picked up by such testing earlier than it would have been previously, the chances of that illness being successfully treated are greater.

Gene testing involves examining a person's DNA – the body's 'building blocks' – which is taken from cells in a sample of their blood or other body fluid, and then looking for some anomaly that equates to known diseases or disorders. With medical science having just completed the extraordinary process of 'mapping' the essence of life in all our DNA, genetic testing is now being used to detect diseases such as cancers years earlier than is possible with conventional preventive medicine. There is still a long way to go, but progress is already being made in both detecting and treating certain cancers. Tests for some rare cancers are in use and the field of genetic testing is evolving all the time:

★ Testing for the so-called BRCA1 gene mutation is already in use. This mutation predisposes someone to hereditary breast cancer and ovarian cancer and is probably responsible for at least 5% of these diseases in younger women. The mutant gene is found in nearly half the families with a high incidence of breast cancer and in over 80% of families with a history of early-onset breast and ovarian cancer. Following the isolation of this gene – and of the associated gene BRCA2 – the increasing use of blood tests in such families can only become more common.

★ A test is in place for the gene that triggers familial adenomatous polyposis coli – a tendency to form hundreds of small polyps inside the large bowel. If not removed, some of these growths can become cancerous and, although the condition can be diagnosed without genetic tests, these will make diagnosis much easier. A family history of bowel cancer is one of the commonest current reasons I refer patients to genetic-testing centres. For example, if I were to see a patient who has a first-degree relative with bowel cancer under the age of 40, my patient would merit colonoscopic checks every five years. If the family history included two first-degree relatives with the condition aged under 50, colonoscopy would begin when the patient was as young as 25–30 and be carried out twice a year up to the age of 65. In addition the patient would be referred to my local genetic-testing centre. Age, degree of relationship and family history are crucial markers for genetic screening in such cases.

★ Following on from this, the set of genes predisposing people to a much more common type of bowel cancer known as hereditary nonpolyposis colon cancer (HNPCC) has been mapped out in high-risk families. As a result, a blood test for this is expected soon.

★ Predictive testing is available for selected families with certain cancers called Wilms' tumours and retinoblastoma.

★ Although no blood tests are currently widely available, the genes have been mapped out for conditions such as leukaemia, thyroid and kidney cell cancers and melanomas.

However, it is important to point out that predictive gene testing will not be commonplace. Such tests will be able to identify no more than a small proportion of people who will develop bowel or breast cancer, for example. Most cancers are not inherited, and the majority of people with cancer – irrespective of whether they have relatives affected with it or not – do not have inherited gene mutations. I expect the 'first wave' of new genetic tests to be aimed at individuals with strong histories of inherited colon or breast cancer over at least two generations. After this, more routine testing over a wider range of illnesses is foreseen. But one thing is certain – we are riding a fast train to a destination where genetic testing for illness is not unusual.

Although genetic testing for inherited diseases is still in its infancy, this area of medicine will explode over the next two decades. If you have a very strong pattern of inherited cancer in your family, you may be able to have an already available test that will indicate whether you are at increased risk.

Beware of sunbeds

Patients often ask me whether tanning beds or booths are dangerous, as they want to 'look fit for summer'. This popular belief that a tan makes you appear young and healthy needs to be balanced against the fact that a tan has nothing to do with health and can in fact be dangerous. Exposure to excessive sunlight has been associated with cancer since as far back as 1894 and most doctors now agree that the use of artificial sun lamps probably doubles our risk of developing certain skin cancers. To understand why, it is important to know why we become tanned when exposed to sunlight.

Ultraviolet light from the sun damages the skin, and this damage causes it to produce a dark pigment called melanin. It is this that causes the skin to darken, and the tan then helps to protect it against further damage from ultraviolet light. However, this protection is by no means perfect and does not preclude further harm. Sun blocks are designed to prevent ultraviolet light damaging the skin, and so when they are used a tan does not occur.

The idea of a sunbed or a tanning booth is to produce much greater amounts of ultraviolet radiation in a given time than the sun does. This allows the user to develop a tan much more quickly than is possible through conventional sunbathing. It also means sunburn can develop much faster, and so a close watch must be kept on the clock.

I know I am never going to stop people wanting a tan – that is human nature – but I always say to patients that not only is pale interesting, it is also healthy. If you plan to use a sunbed or tanning booth and are taking medication, always check with your doctor first. Some drugs can increase the body's reaction to ultraviolet radiation, and while this may not be a problem in sunlight, in the intense ultraviolet light of a sunbed or tanning booth it can be. These drugs include some antibiotics (but not all), diuretics (or 'water tablets'), some oral contraceptives and certain treatments for diabetes and high blood pressure.

My advice on tanning is therefore: don't. But if, after considering the risks, you do go ahead with accelerated tanning, always remember:

★ Wear eye protection. The eyes are especially vulnerable in tanning booths and damage to the front and back of the eye can occur, along with cataracts. Simply closing your eyes or wearing sunglasses is not enough. Always use the special goggles designed for this purpose.

★ Never overdo it. Start with very short exposure times – even if you are tempted to stay longer – and slowly increase the duration.

★ Do not use tanning accelerants such as tanning lotions – these can intensify skin damage.

Remember that having a tan means that your skin has been damaged, and that sunbeds and tanning booths accelerate this process. If you use these, always take precautions and check your skin for new moles or other danger signs.

Fit smoke detectors

Every year hundreds of lives are needlessly lost in domestic fires because no smoke alarm was fitted. Worse, they are sometimes installed and then the batteries are not replaced, and the end result is the same. I have never forgotten just how poignant the sight was when I visited a house gutted by a fire in which the whole family had been killed, and saw a child's teddy bear among the wreckage, along with a smoke detector that had failed to work.

Fortunately, fire services have played a major part in alerting the public to the benefits of smoke alarms, so that an increasing number are bought each year. For most people, these devices are their first line of defence against fire, and the figures on their effectiveness are impressive – if fire breaks out, the smoke alarm, functioning as an early warning system, reduces the risk of dying by nearly 50%. They are the single most important means of preventing house-fire fatalities, and I believe they are the best, as well as the cheapest, safety device you can buy and install to protect yourself, your family and your home.

Install them on every level of your home, as many fatal fires begin late at night or early in the morning, when only the bedrooms are likely to be occupied. They should be fixed either to the ceiling or six to eight inches below it on side walls, since smoke and many deadly gases rise. Installing them at the proper level gives you the earliest possible warning.

Smoke alarms are very easy to maintain. Remember to replace the batteries at least once a year, and if your alarm starts beeping at any other time, put in new batteries and reset it. Dust and debris can interfere with their operation, so keep them clean, vacuuming over and around them regularly. It is very important to test every smoke alarm monthly, and to always use new batteries when replacing dead ones.

You probably spend more time polishing your car each week than you do checking your smoke alarms each year. Which one of these activities is going to save your life?

Smoke alarms are cheap, effective, simple to use and will protect you and your family from the dangers of fire. What further reason do you need for fitting them?

It's my bowels, Doctor

If there is one thing that patients seem to expect from me during a consultation it is an enquiry as to the state of their bowels. I may be having a bad day, look like a mad professor and snarl and grunt, but as long as I ask at some point, 'Bowels all right?', honour is satisfied and another customer walks away happy.

I suppose I am exaggerating slightly, but there is no question in my mind that in this country constipation is a topic of supreme importance to a great many people. There is in fact a great deal of misunderstanding about what constipation means, and many people think they have this problem when their bowel movements are actually regular. My definition of constipation is the passing of small amounts of hard, dry motions fewer than three times a week. What is 'normal' varies from person to person, but anything from three times a day to three times a week is within the normal range, and the key is not to stick slavishly to the belief that unless your bowels open once a day there is something wrong with you.

The removal of waste from our bodies is crucial to good health. You would not keep on lighting a fire that was full of clinker and ash, and after a while it would refuse to light anyway. The same applies to our body, which, as a machine, needs cleaning at regular intervals. Constipation can cause tiredness, abdominal pain, bloating, excessive wind and disorders of the gut, to name but a few common problems, so anything we can do to prevent it is worth recommending.

The most frequent causes of constipation in the Western world are a poor diet and a lack of exercise. Any diet that is low in fibre and high in fat will tend to cause constipation, whereas most people who eat high-fibre foods are not bothered by this problem (although it can affect anyone at any age). With its bulk and soft texture, fibre works to prevent the formation of the dry, hard stools that are so difficult to pass, but the problem is not helped by the consumption of highly processed foods. Fibre alone is not enough, however, since fibre without fluid equals concrete. Drink eight large glasses (eight fluid ounces) of water or fruit juice a day if your fluid intake is poor, and try to avoid tea, coffee and caffeine-containing soft drinks, all of which can dehydrate you.

In older people, a low-fibre diet is responsible for many cases of constipation. Some of them adopt such a diet because false teeth or the loss of teeth makes it necessary to eat blander, softer foods that are low in fibre.

Regular exercise helps to promote regular bowel movements, but this need not be sweaty aerobics – just walking each day is enough. Never ignore the need to go to the toilet, and try to avoid the use of laxatives, which tend to make the problem far worse over time as the body becomes dependent on them to function properly.

Constipation is a problem that has been around for ever, and for many people it is a cause not only of ill health but also of profound embarrassment. Back in the sixteenth century, as he was bowing deep and low to Queen Elizabeth I, the Earl of Oxford – a man apparently prone to constipation – broke wind long and loud. Mortified, he withdrew from the royal court and fled abroad, where he spent several years trying to become anonymous and forget his lack of decorum. When he returned to England he travelled to court to pay his respects to the Queen once more. Before he could say anything, her first words to him were, 'My lord, I had forgot the fart.'

Constipation affects millions of people but is often easily remedied. A high-fibre diet allied to exercise and increased fluid intake is always the starting point in preventing its recurrence.

Take aspirin

I sometimes muse on what I would select if I were exiled to a desert island and allowed to take one item. Although I expect I would end up asking for a case of champagne to be washed up every week, aspirin would be a more sensible choice, especially if I had a history of heart disease.

Aspirin is one of the oldest medications we have, so it is a surprise to many people that it is still often called the 'new wonder drug' in the media. Despite the fact that it is well known for helping to prevent heart attacks and strokes, under half of high-risk patients are actually prescribed the drug and a recent study published in the *British Medical Journal* has estimated that 3,000 deaths could be prevented in the UK, and 40,000 worldwide, if it were given more often. In people who are at increased risk of heart attack or stroke, as well as patients who have already had a heart attack, the blood-thinning properties of aspirin help to improve blood flow through the circulation and so reduce the risk of problems in the future. It can also be used in people with peripheral arterial disease, stable angina or atrial fibrillation (an irregular heart rhythm). There is also exciting work being done at the moment which suggests that aspirin may be of benefit in reducing the growth of prostate cancer by inhibiting a particular body chemical called Cox–II, believed to encourage prostate-cancer cells to grow.

So, should we all be stocking up on aspirin? Well, no. Random long-term use of the drug is medically discouraged because it can contribute to stomach ulcers and bleeding from the gut. For people who are normally healthy but may be slightly more at risk of heart disease for some reason – a family history of heart disease, for example – it remains unclear if the benefits of aspirin outweigh the risks. What is certain, though, is that doctors now need to ensure that aspirin – or a similar blood-thinning drug – is routinely considered for patients who might need it. If you have a history of angina or heart disease, heart attacks or stroke and are not already taking aspirin, ask your doctor if there is any reason why you should not do so. If there is no medical reason for avoiding aspirin, taking it daily could be crucial to your continued good health.

Aspirin tends to be under-used as a long-term preventive treatment against heart attack and stroke. If you have a history of these conditions, discuss with your doctor whether you could benefit from the drug.

Try something smooth and fruity

I am certainly no Bible scholar, but I do remember a quotation from Ecclesiasticus that says, 'Wine is as good as life to man, if it be drunk moderately.' There are many questions about the health benefits of wine. Is it healthy at all? How much is too much? Is it only red wine that is beneficial, and if so, is a vintage Petrus better for you than a youthful Chilean Cabernet?

Before attempting to answer these questions we should acquaint ourselves with the so-called 'French paradox'. This term was coined to explain the lower incidence of heart disease in the French compared with Americans, a difference possibly due in part to the beneficial effect of moderate wine consumption on the heart and circulation. The Henderson pocket guide to explaining this and why wine may have health benefits goes something like the following.

The main point is that the benefits of wine are highly likely to be derived from phenolic compounds, found in high concentrations in grape skins, seeds and stems. These compounds, more often referred to as antioxidants, appear to be beneficial in two ways. First, they help to prevent an unhealthy type of cholesterol (LDL cholesterol) from being laid down as unhealthy plaques that can eventually block blood vessels. Secondly, they reduce the chances of blood clots developing in the body by slightly thinning the blood, especially if wine is drunk during a meal. In addition to these circulatory benefits, there is now evidence to suggest that antioxidants help in the fight against free radicals – naturally occurring and harmful products in our body cells that have been implicated in the development of certain cancers and Alzheimer's disease.

If antioxidants are beneficial, are all wines equally 'healthy'? No, they're not. Red wines in general contain more antioxidants than white (and in this respect they are better than all other alcoholic drinks), but even among red wines there are premier-league vineyards to look out for. Red burgundy, Merlot, Pinot Noir and Chilean Cabernet seem to have the highest levels of the antioxidants resveratrol and flavonol. Wine-pressing techniques in South American wines are more vigorous than in other countries, with the result that the small grapes and their seeds produce a higher concentration of these chemicals. The winemaking process itself is very important in this context, since winemaking uses all parts of the grape and is essentially an anaerobic (airless) activity. It is believed that prolonged exposure to air during open fermentation may destroy naturally occurring antioxidants, and this would explain why grape juice, which is not protected from the air like wine during production, does not appear to have the same beneficial effect as red wine.

The next question to answer is, when should we be drinking? The answer is almost certainly 'with food'. It is this factor which could explain the French paradox, since, despite having a fat-rich diet, the average French person is less likely to die from heart disease than the average Briton. As most wine is drunk with food in France, Spain and Italy – all of which have lower levels of heart disease and higher wine consumption than the UK – it may be the customary pattern of drinking in those countries, as opposed to the binge drinking so often seen in the UK, that makes the important difference. There is, however, an important caveat. This is the fact that it is only in the past two decades or so that the French and British have been consuming equivalent quantities of cholesterol, and it is the French who have been doing the catching up. If the incidence of heart disease in France starts to rise over the next decade, the French paradox may be turned on its head, although many experts believe this is unlikely.

So, you are looking expectantly at your chosen wine while

savouring the aroma of your favourite meal. The next question is, 'How much wine is healthy?' There is little disagreement here, and the current guidelines stand at 14 units per week for women and 21 units per week for men, with one unit equivalent to a 125-millilitre glass of 9%-alcohol wine. Unfortunately for lovers of wine, more is not better, and doubling your intake will not double your health benefits. There is a very fine line between healthy drinking and drinking more than is good for you, with both teetotallers and drinkers of more than four or five units a day having an increased risk of heart disease compared with moderate drinkers. This protective effect increases with age, with the most significant benefits becoming apparent in those older than 60. It must always be stressed, though, that wine is not the panacea for all infirmities. Louis Pasteur may have said, 'Wine is the most healthful and hygienic of beverages', but by itself it cannot fight off the effects of smoking, obesity, raised blood pressure and lack of exercise. However, taken as part of a generally healthy lifestyle, it is quite possibly the most palatable medicine ever invented and that is something I will happily raise a glass of Château Perfectly Fruity to.

Red wine, drunk regularly in small amounts, appears to confer health benefits, whereas drinking none or too much seems to be less healthy. But always remember the Three Ms here – moderation, moderation and moderation.

Sex and gardening and rock and roll

At the launch of yet another gardening show on TV, I am always amused by the notion that's fed to us that this simple pastime is either the new rock and roll or the new sex. Well, I'm sorry, but it isn't. Sex is the new sex and always will be. Gardening may come a close second in terms of health benefits, though, and I often recommend it to patients as a form of regular exercise. Let me explain why.

Innumerable studies have long proved that physical exercise taken on a regular basis reduces your risk of heart disease, early death, stroke, depression, cancer of the large bowel, diabetes and high blood pressure, among many other conditions. Well, gardening combines cardiovascular exercise with flexibility, endurance and muscular strength – just think of all the stretching it entails and combine this with the hard slog of digging and you will get the picture. Real benefits are often obtained in a far more enjoyable manner than by pounding away on a treadmill for hours on end – and paying for the privilege – and these need not be confined to the body either. The mental benefits are obvious too, to the extent that treatment now exists called horticultural therapy, which is based on the therapeutic help obtained from fresh air, sunshine and concentrating on things other than our problems. Simply sitting and looking at trees, plants and flowers has been shown to lower blood pressure, reduce muscle tension and improve well-being by lowering stress levels. You don't even need to be good at it to benefit. But active gardening is even more helpful.

Again and again I find that patients of mine who regularly spend time in their garden lead a more satisfying life, have a well-balanced outlook and feel positive about what they do. I have believed this impression to be true for many years, but it is always nice to have your hunch backed up by some science. According to the Canadian Horticultural Therapy Association, people working in offices without plants were 12% less productive and more stressed than those in plant-filled work areas. More surprisingly, a study of people with Alzheimer's disease found that if they lived in care homes with gardens, the rate of violent incidents reduced by nearly a fifth over two years. At homes without gardens, this rate increased by two thirds over the same period.

There is one further health benefit to be gained at the end of a good day's gardening – a long, hot, relaxing bath. At such times I often recall the words of the great philosopher Bertrand Russell. A friend of his once found him deep in profound thought and asked him why he was so contemplative. Russell replied, 'I think I've made an odd discovery. Every time I talk to colleagues I feel quite sure that happiness is no longer a possibility. Yet when I talk with my gardener, I'm convinced of the opposite.'

Gardening is good for the mind, body and soul, and it doesn't matter whether you are digging a ditch or restoring a subtle-hued flower garden. Even better, it's free and anyone can do it.

Have a healthy flight

Whether you are a frequent flyer or a holidaymaker simply looking forward to two weeks away from the boss, the health risks of flying are more subtle than you might think, although recent media reports about 'economy-class syndrome' have brought these into the public consciousness. The air you breathe during a flight is certainly not of Alpine quality, but before we all jump on the nearest fishing boat instead, there are a great many things we can do to reduce the chances of us leaving a plane sicker than when we boarded it:

★ During a long-haul flight you should always get up and walk about for a few minutes every hour. This reduces the chances of a blood clot developing in the calves as a result of prolonged sitting at altitude. I often see this condition in my patients who have recently travelled, and it is said to affect at least 2,000 people in the UK each year. If you have a history of this problem or suffer from varicose veins, it is sensible to take a daily aspirin several days before flying, as this will help to thin the blood slightly and reduce the risk of blood clots. However, if you have a history of stomach problems or take any other prescription drugs, check with your doctor first.

★ Drink plenty of fluid – and by this I don't mean raid the duty-free trolley. The humidity in a plane can reach 3% – far worse than in the middle of a desert – and alcohol takes effect much more rapidly in a plane than on the ground. Drink water regularly throughout the flight – a minimum of two litres is recommended. This will considerably reduce the problems of headaches, tiredness and jet lag. Some people find that these symptoms are eased by taking vitamins C and E for some weeks before flying, and this effect can be helped by adding the natural supplements ginseng and echinacea.

★ Buy a face mask. This isn't as bizarre as it sounds, and in fact makes very good medical sense. Poor air is an ideal breeding ground for bacteria and promotes person-to-person transmission of illness. (In one well-publicised case a businessman contracted a very nasty pneumonia from a carrier of the same strain of infection who was sitting at the other end of the plane.) Face masks are becoming an increasingly frequent sight on flights, but it is vital to use the right type – an ordinary surgical mask will not work. The present leader in the field is the Aviation Health Institute (AHI) mask, which eliminates the vast majority of transmissible infections and can be used several times before being replaced.

★ Choose where you sit. Air quality varies throughout a plane, with the fresher air being found towards the front, where it is pumped into the passenger area. Before it reaches the back of the plane it has been breathed in and out hundreds of times, so, if your budget will allow it, always fly first rather than economy class.

★ Wear a pair of 'economy-class socks'. These encourage the blood to flow normally through the feet and lower legs.

★ Watch what you eat. Not surprisingly, sitting in a pressurised metal box at 30,000 feet has an effect on any gas that is inside you. This will expand by 20% during a flight, and so it is sensible to avoid gassy drinks or sparkling water while in the air. Any foods that make you feel bloated normally should be avoided if they form part of the in-flight meals.

Keep the meals you eat shortly before flying light and simple – pasta and fruit are ideal. It is better to arrive at your destination slightly hungry and well hydrated than bloated and thirsty.

★ Remember that you are a customer. Some airlines seem to view their passengers as cattle, but you don't have to put up with this. Be aware that cabin staff are obliged to keep the air packs that pull in air from outside the plane working throughout a flight. Airlines are also legally required to carry a set number of oxygen canisters per passenger, and you can ask for one if you are having problems breathing or feel sick.

Taking sensible precautions before and during a flight can turn a potentially unpleasant and unhealthy journey into something to be looked forward to rather than endured. In this way you really can arrive at your destination as healthy as when you set off.

Understand what stress does to you

After writing a book on stress and how to deal with it, I developed something of a reputation as being 'the stress doctor'. Now, this was all fine and dandy until I realised that most of my consultations were on stress-related issues and I was in danger of not seeing any other kind of cases in my surgery. This put me at risk of becoming a bored and stale doctor and – you guessed it – more likely to become stressed. I was able to redress the balance, but it has made me wonder whether I should write a book called *How to Give Millions to Your Doctor and Feel Better* and see what happens.

'Stress' may be a hugely overused word nowadays, but the condition is nevertheless a real problem and it is important to know what effects it can have on the body, because these can directly affect longevity. Apart from the usual symptoms we are all familiar with when we get tense, there are probably five major indicators of stress that I see time and again in my patients. In no particular order, these are:

★ High blood pressure. A good example of this would be a bus driver who has a sedentary job but experiences high levels of stress. Studies have shown that his blood pressure is likely to be higher than that of his more active colleagues, with all the attendant risks, such as heart attacks. In middle-aged people in general, rises in blood pressure caused by stress also predispose them to strokes.

★ A weakened immune system. Stress undoubtedly weakens

our body defences over time if allowed to continue un-checked. It is clear to me that among my college-student patients there are greater numbers of colds and viral illnesses during exam periods. I have also noticed lowered levels of immunity in spouses caring for a seriously ill partner.

★ Muscle weakness. When stress is severe it often causes fatigue and weakness in the muscles.

★ High cholesterol levels. This predisposes to coronary heart disease by 'furring up' the blood vessels that serve the heart.

★ High sugar levels. Stress raises blood sugar levels (which are often pushed up further at the same time by eating sweet, sugary 'comfort' foods) and this can affect the body's pro-duction of insulin. This last problem may be a precursor to diabetes.

The reason I raise these points is to show that stress – especially if chronic or severe – affects the body far more than we may realise, and these effects become more apparent as we age. Dealing with our stress should not be a luxury; it is a necessity if you want to enjoy a long and healthy life. Nowadays so much stress seems to be linked to work, and if you find yourself get-ting steamed up during your working day, ask yourself a simple question: 'Who will remember this in 20 years' time?' The answer is no one, except your body, and we've only got one of those each.

Stress has significant effects on both mind and body, and over the long term it can be highly damaging. If you recognise the symptoms, look for the underlying cause and try to do something about it. You only live once.

Trust me, I'm a doctor

This tip has a double edge to it, since in mentioning it I am effectively inviting an increase in the workload of both myself and my medical colleagues. Nevertheless, the truth is that if more people consulted their doctor early on about worrying symptoms, more of them would have their significant illnesses picked up sooner rather than later. This has the obvious advantage of allowing any necessary treatment to be begun earlier, which in turn increases the likelihood of a cure.

The problem here is that patients need to be somewhat selective about seeking medical advice, otherwise every doctor in the land would be submerged under a tidal wave of coughs, colds and sore throats within a week. For this reason I am certainly not advocating that you hurry along to your doctor at the first sign of any health problem. In fact time is one of the most useful weapons family doctors have in their armoury, since it allows most self-limiting illnesses to do exactly that – limit themselves. However, it is far from sensible to sit on worrying or persistent symptoms for weeks on end in the hope that they will just go away. Diseases such as cancer and heart disease – two of the biggest killers – are no respecters of the calendar or the clock and will thank you for ignoring their warning symptoms.

Very few doctors will have patients who take this advice as literally as the great Field Marshal Montgomery of Alamein. One day, during a sitting of the House of Lords, he was not his usual ebullient self. After a while he calmly turned to the member sitting next to him, and with a completely calm voice and stoical expression, said, 'Do excuse me, but I'm having a coronary thrombosis.' His amazed neighbour watched while he went off to seek medical attention, which confirmed that he had indeed suffered a heart attack.

Why do some people who are worried about their health shy away from seeing their doctor? Apart from anxiety about what may be wrong with them, other common reasons include not being happy with their doctor – unfortunately more common than it should be – and being falsely reassured by family and friends that all is well. And, of course, serious illness can present late without there having been any early warning signs at all, and that is the nature of nature. However, if you experience any such signs, you should bear in mind that any good doctor would far rather be able to reassure a worried patient early than treat a seriously ill one late.

If in doubt, get checked out. It's as simple as that.

20

Don't get angry

Nowadays I seem to see a great many angry people. Much of the time there appears to be very little for them to be cross about, yet they rant and rage as if their whole life depended on it. Which indeed it could do.

Researchers at the University of North Carolina have unveiled new evidence that uncontrolled anger is a threat to health and life. A questionnaire assessing feelings of anger found that people with the highest scores are nearly three times more likely to have a heart attack or die from a sudden cardiac incident than those whose answers show them to be the least anger-prone. At least two other American studies have indicated the same relationship – the Framingham Heart Study, which looked at suppressed anger and heart disease, and one done by the Harvard School of Public Health – but this one is something of a cracker and should be salutary reading to anyone who flies off the handle at the slightest thing.

Nearly 13,000 participants were asked whether they were hot-headed, whether they felt they wanted to hit someone when angered, whether they experienced feelings of frustration and annoyance when no recognition had been given for good work, and so on. Of those questioned, 8% (1,000 people) were ranked at the high end of the scale. In the six-year follow-up period, they were found to be 2.69 times more likely to have a heart attack or suffer sudden death than those ranked lowest. Individuals with moderate feelings of anger were 35% more likely to experience a coronary event. The angriest people were more likely to be cigarette smokers – a major risk factor – but even when smoking and other risk factors, such as diabetes, being overweight and having high cholesterol levels, were taken into account, they were still found to be at higher risk.

If you have a problem with your temper and want to reduce risks to your health, what can you do? Fortunately, there are things that you can do to lower anger and manage it efficiently, starting with looking at what triggers it. Learn also to take 'time out' before you blow. Go for a walk, leave the office, avoid confrontation for the next few minutes – anything – until you calm down.

If self-control doesn't work, you may need to get professional counselling, or to join an anger-management course, both of which help some people. Dealing with anger is currently behind the treatment of other problems, such as anxiety and depression, and intervention strategies and treatments continue to be developed. If you feel that anger is a problem in your life, discuss this with your doctor, because the evidence is growing that being in a rage is bad for our long-term health.

Don't seethe with anger or continually lose your temper. Heart attacks and sudden death are more common in people who habitually act this way than can be explained simply by chance. If your anger is a problem for you, seek professional guidance.

'If you live to the age of a hundred, you have made it because very few people die past the age of a hundred.'

– George Burns

Natural tips

Pins and needles

Acupuncture has been practised for thousands of years in the Far East and has taken hold in the West since the 1970s, especially after a *New York Times* journalist who had his appendix removed while under acupuncture wrote enthusiastically about its pain-relieving properties. Two main forms of acupuncture are used in the West. Practitioners of the traditional Chinese form believe illness arises from an imbalance of the yin and yang 'life forces', and insert needles into various body points to redress this balance. Try as I might to get my head around this idea, my reaction tends to be the same: 'Hmm.'

The other form is more widely practised and focuses on the physical effects a needle can have on the body. Needles are inserted into 'trigger points', or acupoints – sensitive points that are often in areas where nerves enter or leave muscle and tissue. The theory is that if you insert a needle into one of these points, natural endorphin painkillers are released into the bloodstream, as well as natural anti-inflammatory compounds that promote healing.

Acupuncture has many converts, who claim it helps all manner of ills, including back pain – and pain of virtually any kind, in fact – anxiety and stress, high blood pressure and irritable bowel problems. Hard scientific evidence to prove this is scarce, but one study published in the *Royal Society of Medicine Journal* showed that stimulating an acupoint just above the wrist could eliminate nausea in pregnancy, and this work has been successfully reproduced since. Other studies have shown that acupuncture can reduce pain and nausea after surgery, and many doctors now take the view that it makes certain nerves work better by stimulating them. Interestingly, these nerves coincide with traditional Chinese acupoints.

Sceptical about all this, but curious too, I decided to try it for myself. Having been in significant discomfort from a neck problem that seemed resistant to my conventional treatments, I put myself in the hands of an acupuncturist who just happened to be a fellow GP I trusted completely. There was surprisingly little discomfort apart from in those areas where I was having pain anyway, but when I looked at my neck and back in a mirror during the treatment I was amazed to see massive reddening around these areas and nowhere else.

The next day I had no neck pain and have not suffered from this problem since. All in the mind? I think not. My single experience was hardly a scientific trial, but it makes you think, doesn't it?

Many people are convinced that acupuncture cures their pain as well as promoting rapid healing and general well-being. It is safe when carried out by registered practitioners, but always check the qualifications of any acupuncturist with the British Acupuncture Council or the relevant organisation in your own country before accepting treatment.

Use glucosamine

It is not often that I fall off my chair in shock – in my job I consider myself to be pretty unshockable by anything anyone tells me – but I only just stopped myself doing so on receiving a consultant's letter recently. This orthopaedic surgeon, not renowned for his open mind as far as medication of *any* kind is concerned, recommended that I start a patient of mine on glucosamine to treat arthritis, and asked if I knew about it. Well, having been suggesting its use for some years, I was familiar with the name, but what shocked me was that a natural supplement had been accepted by a bastion of the surgical establishment. Anyway, it got me pondering on why glucosamine appears to be so effective for treating arthritis and arthritis-like conditions in so many people. These are a big problem in the UK – almost half the over-65 population will suffer some degree of arthritis in some form. The two best-known examples of the condition are rheumatoid arthritis and osteoarthritis (the 'wear and tear' arthritis), both of which are increasingly prevalent. However, many sufferers are reluctant to use prescription drugs exclusively to relieve their symptoms.

This is where glucosamine comes in. A natural constituent of cartilage, it has been shown to stimulate the body's production of connective tissue. In mainland Europe it has been used to treat arthritis since the 1980s and it does appear to be genuinely low in side effects, which is more than can be said for the conventional anti-arthritis medications many doctors in the UK prescribe. The hard science is somewhat equivocal, however, since although study results are generally positive, they are not so thorough that I could call them conclusive. Nevertheless, some specialists – including my new best friend – now believe that glucosamine preparations not only relieve the symptoms of arthritis but may actually halt the deterioration so commonly seen. If taken in conjunction with another supplement, chondroitin, it may work even more effectively, as chondroitin attracts more fluid into joint spaces, thus oiling them more effectively.

Glucosamine needs to be taken for at least a month – in some cases for up to three months – before the benefit becomes apparent. How effective it really is may become clearer after a five-year study now being undertaken in America which is looking at its long-term use in conjunction with chondroitin. Smaller studies are also in progress, but if you don't want to wait until these results are available, you will do yourself no harm by starting to take glucosamine now.

Glucosamine, like chondroitin, is becoming increasingly recognised as an effective natural treatment for joint pain and arthritis. Side effects are rare and it is not foreign to the body.

3

Get your antioxidants

What are antioxidants? Well, these interesting little things are probably as crucial to our long-term health as any dietary supplement or natural health food you can find. In essence, these are the vitamins A, C and E, plus selenium (a mineral) and a group known as the carotenoids. Carotenoids, of which beta-carotene is the most commonly found, are pigments that add colour to many fruits and vegetables.

Antioxidants are thought to be effective in helping to prevent chronic disease and so are extremely important because they slow cell destruction in the body by neutralising 'free radicals', which cause this damage. Free radicals are found in pollution (both atmospheric and chemical) and cigarette smoke, and it has been postulated that it is their presence in the second that gives heavy smokers a much more 'lined' and aged appearance than non-smokers of the same age. Even more importantly, some doctors believe that cancer changes in cells may initially be triggered in part by the damage that free radicals inflict on them.

We are often very good at doing the 'outside' stuff in our efforts to slow down the effects of ageing. We try to get more sleep, we drink lots of water, we exercise regularly and we slap on lots of the latest anti-wrinkle cream at vast expense (well, not me personally, you understand). However, we tend to forget that our cells are fuelled from the inside and that what we should be doing is loading our bodies with lots of antioxidant-rich foods. The fresher the better here, and organic too, if possible. Good examples of such foods are:

★ Fruits such as peaches, grapes, apples, berries, bananas and citrus fruits, and their fresh juices.

★ Mushrooms and nuts.

★ Dark-green, leafy vegetables, celery, onions, beets, carrots and broccoli.

★ Baked potatoes.

So, shouldn't we all be taking in super-doses of antioxidants? Well, not quite. There is still much debate as to which groups of people, if any, benefit from taking antioxidant supplements. Some studies have shown that smokers with diets high in carotenoids have a lower rate of lung cancer than smokers with a low carotenoid intake, but this evidence is cancelled out by studies suggesting that some beta-carotene takers, primarily smokers, actually had higher death rates. Other research has suggested that diets high in carotenoids may also be associated with a decreased risk of breast cancer.

Therefore, rather than regarding everyone as a potential beneficiary of antioxidants, it makes more sense to say that the elderly (especially those with a poor food intake), frequent aspirin users, heavy drinkers, smokers and people with impaired immune systems may benefit from taking antioxidant supplements daily. But such supplements should never be used as substitutes for a fresh, healthy, well-balanced diet, and we must not forget we can actually over-supplement our bodies, taking much more than the recommended daily amount of certain vitamins and minerals. Vitamins A and E are fat-soluble, which means that excess amounts are stored in the liver and fatty tissues, instead of being quickly removed from the body. I have actually seen a patient walk into my surgery who was a vivid orange colour because of eating too many carrots. Supplement by all means, but keep it sensible.

Antioxidants are a powerful tool in reducing the harmful effects of free radicals on our bodies. They are found in fresh fruits and vegetables, and appear to help to reduce the risk of heart disease and cancer.

Free the coenzyme Q_{10}

During my travels as a medical writer I run into all sorts of people who jot down words on health for a living, and among these are experts on natural or 'alternative' treatments. When, rather mischievously, I ask them what is the supplement they would take themselves if they could choose only one, the majority say the same thing – CoEnzyme Q_{10}. At this point I used to smile knowingly, mutter, 'Ah, of course', and go away wondering what on earth they were talking about. Well, now I know, and it's good stuff.

CoQ_{10}, as it is called by those in the know, was discovered in the 1950s as a fat-soluble substance that occurs naturally in plant and animal tissue. Research subsequently showed it to be crucial in the production of cell energy, and so it is an energy provider at a very basic cellular level. Although it occurs naturally in our bodies, and we have large concentrations in our hearts, liver, kidney and pancreas, it is sensible to have a diet rich in it to make sure that we do not become deficient in this most important of coenzymes.

Dietary sources of CoQ_{10} include lean meat, fish, leafy vegetables, grape seed and vegetable oils and soya beans. It is now available as a supplement, but it is best gained from food. Also, because cooking can destroy it, the way to derive the maximum benefit is to eat raw foods that contain it. Surprisingly, exercise also increases our CoQ_{10} levels – another argument for staying active in old age.

So many and varied are the health benefits attributed to CoQ_{10} that I doubt they can all be true, but there are areas where the evidence is significant. Our heart and cardiovascular system can be improved by its use and patients suffering from valvular heart disease and cardiomyopathies often say to me how much better they feel when taking it. It is said to help to open up the circulation in and around the heart and so lower blood pressure by reducing resistance to blood flow.

Our immune system is another area where CoQ_{10} is believed to be beneficial, in protecting our cells from free radical damage. If this claim is true, use of the supplement will have the further effect of helping with heart disease and even some cancers. Most people seem to feel some benefit to their energy levels if they take a daily dose of about sixty milligrams, increasing this to ninety milligrams when stressed or particularly fatigued. As a doctor, I am rather reassured by the fact that there have been few, if any, reports of adverse side effects resulting from use of CoQ_{10}, for we must never forget the medical maxim 'First, do no harm.'

CoEnzyme Q_{10} is a very popular supplement and works by producing energy in every cell of the body. It both strengthens the immune system and revitalises the body by boosting circulation and increasing tissue oxygenation.

Try echinacea

One of the world's most popular herbal treatments, echinacea has been used for centuries. There are records of its use by native American Indians, who found it beneficial for a number of conditions, including snake bite, toothache and sore throat. In Britain it was used by quacks to treat syphilis, typhoid and gangrene, though, not surprisingly, it had little effect on such conditions.

Many studies have been done to test the efficacy of this plant, whose main benefit appears to be that it boosts the body's immune system. The root and flowers contain a chemical called echinacosides and the leaves contain the polysaccharide heteroxylan. All parts of the plant are used, and the effects are linked to its ability to help to prevent the formation in the body of an enzyme called hyaluronidase. This is thought to break down the body's natural barrier between our cells and infectious organisms such as viruses and so make us more vulnerable to the effects of infection. For this reason I find echinacea extremely helpful in patients who are run down or who suffer from repeated infections or chronic fatigue. Cancer patients are also said to benefit by having their immune systems boosted by echinacea, although I do not routinely recommend it for this, preferring to use it to help to fight common infections instead. Extracts from the root of the plant help to reduce the symptoms of colds, flu and other viral infections and it can also be used topically on the skin, sometimes combined with an antifungal cream. I have seen psoriasis and eczema improved considerably in patients using topical echinacea ointment, and simple abrasions, burns and cuts too. Gargled, it can relieve symptoms of a sore throat, and at the very least it should be part of anyone's natural pharmacy.

A very important point to remember about echinacea is that it should not be taken continuously, otherwise the immune system may become over-stimulated. Therefore I always recommend that patients take it for one month and then stop for four to six weeks before using it again. Echinacea is available in a number of forms, including capsules, ointments and lozenges. It seems to be possible to use it with both conventional medication and any other herbal supplements, but always check with your doctor before starting to take it.

Echinacea is one of nature's great natural healers, helping to reduce the effects of infections and strengthening the immune system. Take it on an intermittent basis for the best and safest effect.

Understand free radicals

Free radicals are not some kind of anarchist group, but in fact are far more dangerous and certainly more common. They are the normal by-products of our cell metabolism, and as such we cannot ignore them. Unfortunately, they can damage cells to the point where, if the body fails to neutralise them, their effect will prove fatal. We now have increasing evidence that in the majority of serious illnesses most of the major damage is done by free radicals. For example, during a heart attack, when the supply of oxygen and glucose is cut off to our heart muscles, vast quantities of free radicals are formed and it is these that cause the real damage to heart cells. Inflammation of any kind will also produce them, but it is debatable whether it is the free radicals themselves that are the cause of the inflammation rather than the effect, making conditions such as rheumatoid arthritis worse. Every second of every day the body's cells are under attack by free radicals, but fortunately we can fight back and give ourselves the best chance of not suffering any consequences from their efforts.

In fact the body itself does a lot of the hard work here. We produce large amounts of an enzyme called superoxide dismutase, which converts free radicals to hydrogen peroxide. Because the latter is potentially toxic, it is in turn broken down into water and oxygen by two other enzymes, catalase and glutathion peroxidase. The body is instructed to make these enzymes by its genetic code, and those who know how selective the evolutionary process is understand that nature would not do something like this unless there was a very good reason. The reason is that free radicals are bad for us.

Our salvation also lies in the shape of antioxidants. In general, the damage that is done is caused by the process of oxidation, and attacks on our cells by free radicals are known as oxidative stress. Antioxidants limit this damage. Two of the most effective are vitamins C and E. Vitamin E, also known as tocopherol, is particularly important as it dissolves in fat and most free radical damage is done to fat-containing molecules. Vitamin C, however, is soluble in water and so gets distributed to all parts of the body. The two vitamins together are a powerful combination.

Once again it's appropriate to emphasise that the better the quality of the fuel we put in our own engine, the greater the benefit to our health. A diet that contains a regular daily intake of fresh fruit and vegetables, both of which are rich in antioxidants, is the best way to help the body in its constant battle against the damaging effects of free radicals.

To reduce the damage done to your body by free radicals, eat plenty of fresh fruit and vegetables, don't smoke and supplement your diet with vitamins C and E.

What would I need ginseng for?

Ginseng is a most interesting herb, but for many people it is associated exclusively with anecdotal reports of its aphrodisiac qualities. While this supposed benefit is rooted in myth rather than fact, ginseng does have many other properties that can enhance both the quality and the length of our lives. These have been proven in a wide variety of places, including in space, when ginseng was used by Soviet cosmonauts instead of amphetamines. Olympic athletes used to take ginseng regularly to boost their performance on the track, before sensitive drug testing made its use inadvisable. Most people who take it now do so because it stimulates their performance when tired and reduces fatigue.

It is often not realised that different types of ginseng are on sale, most of them based on Asian, American or Siberian forms of the herb. I stopped counting the different forms, dosages and combinations of ginseng in a health supermarket when I got to the 100 mark.

But what is its secret? Well, its roots contain natural compounds called saponins. Found in many plants and herbs, these have been shown to have potential in preventing heart and circulatory disease, as well as inhibiting the formation of limpid peroxides in heart muscle. Some saponins have beneficial effects on the immune system and may even have anti-tumour properties. Laboratory and human studies show that patients who take ginseng consistently report an improvement in energy, well-being and mental clarity.

I tell my patients to take 100 milligrams of ginseng extract four times a week in a cyclical fashion – two weeks on, two off – but I always advise them to look out for side effects. The main side effect I see is insomnia, especially with the Asian form of ginseng. High doses interfere with sleep, and can slowly accumulate in the system over time. This is why regular breaks from the herb are advisable, and also why it should not really be taken with other stimulant supplements. However, ginseng remains a safe and effective natural herb that is a good energiser and one which improves general well-being.

Ginseng comes in many forms. Asian ginseng tends to stimulate, American ginseng tends to calm and Siberian has an effect that is between these two. Watch out for insomnia when using any form of ginseng, and to achieve maximum benefit take it in short courses rather than continuously.

Gingko biloba?

The gingko tree is most commonly found in China, where for almost 3,000 years it has been used to treat various ailments, and it is from the tree's fruits and seeds that gingko biloba is derived. This natural remedy has long been said to be helpful in treating depression, tinnitus, headache and problems with memory, and it was thought that this was due to its effect on the circulation and the fact that it is an antioxidant. However, an American study in 1997 put the cat among the pigeons when it suggested that it might be of use in treating the symptoms of Alzheimer's disease. Although the report was careful to say that gingko biloba would have no effect whatever on preventing this type of dementia, it has triggered further work into whether there is a case for using it more widely. Germany has taken the plunge and suggested that a daily dose of 240 milligrams of gingko biloba extract should be taken by patients with Alzheimer's disease, but there is still not enough information to recommend its widespread use.

Three important tests were performed in the American study. In the first, participants with mild to moderate dementia of an Alzheimer's type showed a slight improvement in mental processes such as knowing and learning. Secondly, their carers scored them as being slightly improved in mood and social behaviour after taking gingko biloba. Thirdly – and more frustratingly – doctors using 'assessment of change' tests reported no improvement. Clearly, much more work is needed, but results are expected soon which will show whether gingko biloba does in fact offer real medical benefits.

I warn patients against taking gingko biloba without checking with me first, since it is not without risks. Preparations vary in strength and effectiveness, and people taking blood-thinning medication, and those who have problems with their circulation

or blood clotting, should be wary of using it. It is also important to remember that symptoms suggestive of Alzheimer's disease may be caused by other conditions, including dehydration,
depression, thyroid problems and poor nutrition. However, if
Alzheimer's has been confirmed and there are no reasons why
gingko biloba cannot be taken, then it will do no harm and may
even improve symptoms in the short term.

**Gingko biloba has been used in the East for centuries and
early reports suggest that it may have a beneficial effect on
some patients with Alzheimer's disease. However, it will not
prevent this condition occurring in the first place, and
more research is needed.**

Don't ignore St John's Wort

I am allergic to medical quackery and the latest fads – they make me break out in sudden attacks of common sense. However, good medicine should take account of what works for people, and if an unconventional treatment is backed up with medical evidence, so much the better. This is the situation I find myself in when suggesting to patients with severe stress or very mild depression that, instead of taking a prescription drug from me, they first try the herbal medication St John's Wort, or hypericum,

This herb, named after the day on which it is said to flower every year, has recently become popular among the public in the UK, and a recent study published in the *British Medical Journal* appears to support the view that its use is beneficial for the problems I've just mentioned. I have found this reassuring, since St John's Wort is one of only half a dozen natural remedies I routinely suggest to patients with certain medical conditions, and I have been doing so for some years now. It seems to me that, whenever possible, patients are increasingly keen to try non-prescription treatments in the first instance. The medical profession cannot stick its collective head in the sand and hope that this trend will go away, since it is obvious that it will not.

St John's Wort is an excellent example of the benefits and drawbacks of natural treatments, its most evident advantage being that its side effects are much milder than those of conventional antidepressants. The main ones quoted to me are a skin rash when exposed to the sun, slight nausea and dizziness, sleep disturbances and headache. The drug should not be taken with conventional antidepressants or the contraceptive pill, but, even so, few people seem to discontinue their treatment in comparison with users of antidepressants, which can have marked side effects. Another factor is cost; like many natural treatments, St John's Wort is not cheap, although I have noticed people buying it readily spending three times the cost of a standard prescription. In Germany, the preparation is available from doctors on prescription, and is prescribed nearly ten times more commonly than Prozac, but in the UK this level of usage is some distance in the future.

It is important to realise that St John's Wort is not a panacea for unhappiness and that it will not prove effective in any case of depression beyond the very mild. Nevertheless, it would seem to be that rare breed of treatment that is both natural and has some scientific evidence behind it to show that it works. If you are thinking about using St John's Work, consult your doctor if you are already taking other medication or if you are depressed, since close monitoring of this condition is absolutely essential.

If you suffer from significant stress or occasional mild depression, discuss the possibility of taking St John's Wort with your doctor. This is alternative medicine that really can help.

Water, water everywhere

Drink more water and you will feel better. There – medical advice doesn't come much more basic than this, and yet many of us live our lives in a state of chronic dehydration. You would not choose to run your car with barely any oil in it, and yet this is in effect what millions of us are doing to our bodies every day of the week.

Let's look at some basic facts. When we are born almost 97% of our body is made up of water, and the proportion is still some 75% in adulthood. Our brain cells are mainly water and even our teeth have a water content of 10%. Every single cellular function in the body is in some way linked to the body's fluid levels, and at any time about 15% of our total body water is stored in our muscles. Our blood and our cancer-fighting immune systems require water to flush waste products out of cells and to transport nutrients and vital amino acids to them. Healthy cells work by absorbing nutrients from the water that bathes them, and although we can survive for days without food, most of us will be knocking at the gates of St Peter if we have gone without water for a similar length of time. Even a 2% body dehydration is said to cause energy levels to drop by one fifth.

So what should we do about our water intake? The conventional advice is to drink at least eight large glasses (eight fluid ounces) of water each day, since this is said to help to protect the body against disease, promote healthy bowel and kidney function and keep the normal workings of the body at optimum efficiency. This figure is the best estimate of how much water most of us tend to lose over a 24-hour period through normal activities. In an ideal world the best water to choose would be distilled water. This is partly because tap water is often contaminated by pollutants such as pesticides and nitrates, and also because bottled water is not always the squeaky-clean fluid its manufacturers would like us to believe. In fact many so-called 'spring' waters undergo few, if any, checks for pollutants. A carbon-based water-purification filter can be easily fitted to a drinking-water supply system to remove any heavy metals and bacteria, and will repay the cost of installation many times over in health benefits. Filter jugs are also available, but while using one of these is better than not filtering drinking water at all, it may not eliminate heavy metals and bacteria.

One point about water that is often forgotten is that drinking it before eating can actually help with weight loss. If you don't believe me, try drinking water steadily through the day but especially 20 minutes before eating a meal, and watch the weight gradually come off.

Remember that tea, coffee and caffeine-containing soft drinks can dehydrate the body, since they act as diuretics, forcing out fluid. Many dehydrated patients of mine, presenting with typical symptoms such as headaches and fatigue, believe they are drinking enough when in fact they take only these types of drink, with the result that their fluid intake does not keep pace with their output.

Dehydration affects millions of people, yet it is easy to forget that water is crucial for a healthy body and mind. Drink distilled or filtered water or fresh fruit juices rather than caffeine-based drinks if possible.

Exercise – you know it makes sense

The therapeutic benefits of regular physical activity have been known for years, with study after study showing that it increases longevity while decreasing morbidity and mortality from a wide range of diseases. I sometimes think that if exercise were a pill, it would be the most powerful medication known to humans. So why should it be so good for us? My personal favourite reasons are:

★ It detoxes our bodies of the neurotransmitters, hormones and nutrients that are activated, released and metabolised by stress. Regular exercise is useful in removing the by-products of stress by providing the opportunity to simulate the fighting or running dictated by the 'fight or flight' reaction triggered by stress.

★ It acts as a healthy outlet for anger and hostility, those most caustic of emotions.

★ Certain forms of exercise, such as jogging or swimming, require a fairly consistent repetitive motion that can alter your state of consciousness. The physiological effects of regular participation in these activities are very similar to what happens when you practise meditation, and indeed the breathing and movement involved may be partly responsible for the feelings of calmness and tranquillity that some claim are induced by exercise.

★ For some people exercise is an escape from their daily

pressures, while others use this time to reflect on issues of importance or for creative problem-solving.

★ During stress, muscles contract and lose their normal resting tone. Bouts of physical activity allow muscles to work, thereby releasing stored energy and allowing muscle groups to return to their normal resting potential.

★ Catecholamines, including endorphins, have been shown to increase during physical activity of twenty to thirty minutes or more. Chemically similar to opiates, these morphine-like substances have been shown to provide an analgesic effect and promote a sense of euphoria – the so-called 'runner's high'. This occurrence is so significant that some have suggested that exercise is a more effective treatment for clinical depression than psychotherapy or antidepressants.

★ Exercise has been shown to be very effective in helping some individuals to fall asleep easily and sleep more soundly – a very healthy way to treat insomnia.

Don't forget that your body is designed to be exercised just as any engine is designed to be started and run. We may live in the twenty-first century but we still have the same body design as our ancestors did tens of thousands of years ago.

We all know that exercise is good for us. But, beyond the obvious improvements to your cardiovascular system, there are a great many other reasons for making it a regular feature of your life.

Get your share of vitamin E . . .

In a society where a correct diet is increasingly regarded as crucial to health, it is ironic that medical students receive very little formal training in nutrition. I certainly never looked at the role of vitamins, minerals and supplements, yet as a family doctor I come across health issues linked to diet time and time again. It was Hippocrates, the father of medicine, who said, 'Let food be thy medicine', and who believed that diet should be the first step in treating poor health before any medicine is considered.

In our supposedly more enlightened times we more often reach for the prescription pad, but diet remains critically important and eating correctly can be far healthier than resorting to medication. Nutritional supplements are extremely helpful for some people, and although a great deal of rubbish is spouted about the benefits of many of these, this is not the case with vitamin E, which is used as an anti-ageing pill, a heart-protecting pill and a cancer preventer. There are several key points to consider about this vitamin:

★ Over the past decade a steady body of evidence has slowly accumulated to show the value of vitamin E in protecting the heart against disease. As an antioxidant it helps to protect the heart cells from the harmful effects of our metabolism and some doctors are now recommending it to patients as a routine treatment. Laboratory and animal studies suggest that vitamin E helps to reduce the risk of coronary artery disease in a number of ways. First, it inhibits the oxidation of LDL ('bad') cholesterol. Oxidation makes LDL more likely to promote the build-up of fatty plaque in coronary artery walls (atherosclerosis). Secondly, vitamin E may also reduce the blood's ability to clot, thus lowering the risk of heart attacks. Finally, it may help to reduce inflammatory processes, and inflammation of the coronaries has been linked with coronary artery disease.

★ It may boost our immune system. If you are prone to recurring infections, a daily supplement of 200–400 iu may help to prevent this.

★ While vitamin E is no substitute for a healthy diet rich in the antioxidants provided by fresh fruit and vegetables, a daily supplement will do no harm at all, and probably some good, to the elderly and those who, for whatever reason, have a poor diet.

In short, vitamin E is up there in the top five of Henderson's Best Supplements, along with echinacea, glucosamine, St John's Wort and CoEnzyme Q_{10}.

If you have heart disease, are under severe stress or eat a poor diet, vitamin E is a nutritional supplement that has stood the test of time.

. . . and vitamin C

'Vitamin C is really good for you.'
  'How do you know?'
  'Well, it just is, isn't it?'
  This is the sort of conversation I can have when patients talk to me about whether or not they should be taking vitamin C. There is probably more myth and half truth surrounding this nutritional supplement than any other, despite the fact that it is one of the most investigated. Its rise to public awareness probably began back in the early 1970s with the publication of *Vitamin C and the Common Cold*, by the great scientist and biochemist Linus Pauling. In this book Pauling recommended that we should be taking very large doses of vitamin C (around one gram – much more than had been recommended previously) to ward off colds. This went down like a lead balloon in most scientific quarters, where it was held that since vitamin C is a water-soluble vitamin, the more you took the more you simply passed in your urine. So, not only was your wee full of vitamins, but it was also an expensive way of doing nothing for your health. However, Pauling stuck to his guns and continued to take mega-doses until his death in his early nineties. Perhaps there was something to it after all.

  Thirty years later this topic still divides the medical profession. Pauling appears to have been both right and wrong. Many subsequent double-blind clinical studies have found there to be no consistent evidence that taking high doses of vitamin C reduces the number of colds we get. However, many did find that there was a 25% reduction in the length and severity of the cold symptoms, so, while vitamin C won't stop a cold hitting you, it might make you feel a little better when one does.

  How much is enough? Well, you will not go far wrong by

taking 250 milligrams per day, and increasing this temporarily if you have a cold or flu. One of the rationales behind taking vitamin C daily is that it has other health benefits, such as giving protection against heart disease (it is an antioxidant and so protects the body against free radicals, which harm cells) and improving the body's ability to heal itself. A lack of vitamin C causes scurvy – the old curse of sailors – in which gums bleed, teeth fall out, wounds don't heal and bruises occur very easily.

People who smoke need more vitamin C than others do, and good dietary sources include citrus fruits, tomatoes, peppers, broccoli and potatoes. However, there are two reasons why taking continuous mega-doses may not be a good idea. First, it may interfere with the absorption of other vitamins such as B12, and, secondly, it may predispose to the development of low levels of vitamin C once these large doses cease.

Vitamin C is undoubtedly good for you. It helps to protect against heart disease and may reduce the duration and severity of colds. But you do not need massive doses to gain its benefits – more is not necessarily better.

Try a hands-on approach

For my fortieth birthday recently I took myself off to the best hotel in London, made a phone call and was soon in a darkened room with a very pleasant and completely unknown lady in a uniform. After agreeing with her what I wanted and parting with some money, I took my clothes off, lay down on a bed and proceeded to have an extremely pleasant hour, only broken by the occasional need for me to change position.

This hour of massage – what else did you think I was talking about? – left me feeling relaxed and refreshed, feelings that persisted for several days before my muscles began knotting up again with the stresses of modern living. Not only was I generally relaxed, but areas of my body which have always caused me problems, such as my neck and shoulders, were feeling completely pain-free and supple for the first time that I could remember. My therapist pointed out that the knots in my left shoulder muscles were as bad as she had seen and she wondered aloud whether this was a referred problem from a disc in my lower back, but I was completely unaware of any such problem and so dismissed the idea. Nine months later I was on an operating table having major spinal surgery on – you guessed it – a long-standing lower disc problem that was already there when I was being attended to by my masseuse.

For thousands of years massage has been a valid tool in helping the healing process, and the great Hippocrates wrote: 'The physician must be experienced in many things, but assuredly in rubbing. For rubbing can bind a joint that is too loose, and loosen a joint that is too rigid.' Some 1,500 years later, in the eleventh century, the Arab physician Avicenna noted that the object of massage was to 'disperse the effete matters found in the muscles and not expelled by exercise'.

Massage can improve our sense of well-being at any age – how many times have we said to our children, 'Let's rub it better'? – but at no time do we receive less touch than in the later decades of our lives. Cold and stiff limbs and joints can be improved by simple massage and, so long as there is no active inflammation present at the time, even arthritic joints can be eased by gently stretching them to their point of resistance and within pain limits.

Although nothing can take the place of a wise diet and an active lifestyle, massage can readily help to combat many problems associated with ageing. High blood pressure can be reduced, recovery from depression may be speeded up and simple loneliness – a factor that many people forget but which affects the health of countless people – alleviated. The circulation and joints benefit especially, and skin suppleness and muscle tone may improve too.

It is sad to think that now, when we know more about the human body than ever before, the simplest and most old-fashioned anti-stress agent known to man is often ignored – human touch.

Massage is one of the best ways of relaxing. Apart from de-stressing us – with all the benefits that this brings – it can help our joints, circulation and skin and reduce pain.

Float away your stress

This is a tip I readily confess to never having tried, but patients of mine who have simply swear by it, and who am I to argue with anyone who chooses to lie in a sealed tank of water in complete darkness? Many devotees say they feel as if they are going back to the womb and a state of utter and profound relaxation, but my view is more prosaic – it sounds like a great way of getting away from the world for an hour or so.

The idea behind flotation tanks is a simple one, and one that dates back to the 1950s, when an American scientist was investigating what happened to the brain when all external stimuli were removed. He believed that if all such stimuli ceased to exist, the body would have to switch off and go into a coma-like state. However, we now know that this does not happen and that the brain continues to process information and work in a creative manner.

A flotation tank is basically a darkened fibre-glass container filled with salty water that is at skin temperature and less than one foot deep. You need not be in total darkness unless you want to, since a light switch is in the tank (as well as an alarm button, in case of panic), and there is enough space above you to make it unlikely that you will feel claustrophobic. Most flotation sessions last for an hour or so, and this allows you to concentrate fully on relaxing and breathing deeply and slowly – which in turn promotes relaxation. Because your body feels weightless, as well as profoundly relaxed, the brain waves are slowed, which leads to an increase in the brain in mood-lifting endorphins.

Flotation is said to encourage many things. including quicker recovery from injury, creativity in writers and artists, and improved sporting achievement. All these are aided by the body's being able to shut down and heal itself, which is essentially what a flotation session enables it to do. If I ever get the time I just might try this as a means of de-stressing, but all methods such as this come back to the same thing – relaxing is good for you, and we should all do it more often. The less stress we have in our lives, the better our bodies feel for it.

Flotation works for many people and can undoubtedly help to reduce anxiety and stress. Anything that does this is to be recommended, although this remedy will not be to everyone's taste.

Osteopathy – click, crack, crunch

Osteopathy is a therapy that I often recommend to my patients, and is one that they are often happy to accept. The theory is a simple one – our organs are supported by our bones and muscles, and if these are all correctly in line, then everything is hunky-dory. However, stress, poor posture or injury can alter this alignment and so cause pain or impaired nerve function, as well as affecting our general well-being. The aim of osteopathy is to ease any muscle tension and restore bone and joint function to normal, so that the body can heal itself properly. Osteopaths believe that our body framework is not simply 'scaffolding' but is crucial in maintaining good health, and will be concerned as to why there should be a fault in this in the first place. They will look at all possible reasons for the problem, including lifestyle and mental health.

People are sometimes confused about the difference between osteopaths and chiropractors, since they work in a similar manner. Chiropractors usually concentrate on manipulating joints that are not correctly aligned, whereas osteopaths do more soft-tissue treatment, with the aim of relaxing muscles and so improving joint mobility. There are a few points to remember when consulting an osteopath:

★ Any osteopathic treatment will be formulated to meet your individual needs and adapted as treatment progresses.

★ Always use an osteopath registered with the UK Council of Osteopaths or the appropriate approved college in other countries.

★ Osteopathic procedures range in strength from gentle manipulation of the joints to sudden, high-velocity movements that are painless but which can cause dramatic 'clicks' or 'cracks' as joints are repositioned.

★ In some cases one session, usually lasting up to an hour, is enough, but the average treatment is three to six sessions.

★ Some stiffness after treatment is common for a couple of days, and during this time it is advisable not to do any strenuous activity.

★ Do not have osteopathy if you have bone cancer or bone infections, and avoid vigorous manipulation if you have badly prolapsed spinal discs.

I find osteopathy very effective for people with whiplash injuries of the neck, and for those who spend a lot of time working on a computer and as a result develop poor posture, with consequent stiffness and pain in the neck and shoulders. These and low back pain are the problems for which osteopathy is most commonly used.

Osteopathy is one of the complementary treatments most widely used in the West, and is especially useful in treating back pain and neck or shoulder stiffness. Always use an approved practitioner.

Try homeopathy

When discussing homeopathy, and indeed natural medicine in general, I tend to ask 'Will it work?' rather than 'Will it harm?' A recent study undertaken to find out what support there is among GPs for homeopathy found that only 10% of those who responded had never recommended or referred patients for any complementary therapy, while the majority had actually suggested homeopathy to a patient at some time. In fact half the GPs wanted further training in complementary therapy in order to broaden their working knowledge of this area of medicine. Many similar studies have also suggested that there is a greater desire among doctors to learn more about homeopathy and the other branches of natural treatments than there was just 20 years ago.

However, nothing is ever this simple, and homeopathy is no exception. To my medical way of thinking, there is a big fly in the homeopathic ointment, and it takes the shape of scientific analysis. To understand why conventional medicine – which is becoming more open-minded in many quarters – remains to be won over by homeopathy, we must first look at why it is said to work in the first place. It is a system that revolves around the theory that 'like cures like', so that a poison that is causing symptoms of an illness in an individual can then be used to treat those same symptoms. Homeopaths believe that the body is integrated by a 'vital force' that maintains its normal healthy functioning, and that illness occurs when this force is put under strain. Symptoms of illness are viewed as the body healing itself by using its own natural powers, and homeopathy aims to stimulate this self-healing process. Substances are therefore diluted many times – to the point where virtually no molecules of the substance remain in the remedy – but homeopaths believe that such preparations still have sufficient 'likeness' to the illness to stimulate self-healing by the body.

From the point of view of the medical establishment, this is where it all starts to go shaky. While many doctors accept the fact that small quantities of a chemical substance can alter physiological activity in the body, it is hard to see the logic in using a substance so diluted that it is said to be the equivalent of a pinch of salt in the Atlantic Ocean. The theory that electromagnetic 'footprints' of the original substance remain in the diluted mixture, to which the body then responds – the so-called 'water memory' theory – is viewed as risible and completely against all the laws of science by most medical experts. Many doctors feel that any beneficial effects of homeopathy that are described are due in part to a combination of the placebo effect of taking any medication – conventional or alternative – and the considerable time given by homeopathic practitioners to their clients. This may involve consultations of an hour or more, during which close attention is paid to factors such as emotions and the personal beliefs of that individual. Most other complementary therapies also have the benefit of being able to let the client discuss their problems at length – something that many doctors know can be of immense benefit to their patients but which they are simply unable to provide when working to the customary tight schedule.

So, can homeopathy be of benefit to some of those patients whom conventional medicine appears to be unable to help? Undoubtedly. Are doctors as a group slowly recognising that many patients now view homeopathy and other 'natural' treatments as their initial preferred option? Probably. Is there any logical basis in science why homeopathy should work and that a 'vital force' holds our health and well-being together? Not to me. However, you cannot ignore the fact that if a treatment makes someone feel better it is probably doing them some good, and I know a great many very elderly patients who swear that their longevity is due to regular homeopathy. Who is to say they are wrong? The best doctors I know start with a closed prescription pad and an open mind, but not one that is blind to science.

Homeopathy seems to work for a great many people despite the fact that the medical establishment views it with scepticism. If it works for you, it works for you.

Understand
mitochondria

I had forgotten all about mitochondria until I started researching
this book, and then it brought back memories of dusty biology
lessons in my teens, grappling with the finer points of cell struc-
ture. In truth, most of what I learned at school, along with a huge
chunk of my training at medical school, has been supremely useless in my career. However, by understanding a little about what
drives our body's energy system we can try to do something about
those times when we feel exhausted and stressed out.

You cannot see mitochondria unless you use a microscope,
though if you can imagine what wood lice look like from above
you will not be far wrong. They have an outer and inner layer,
with folds, known as 'cristae', where the energy production line
is located. Mitochondria work by producing ATP (adenosine
triphosphate) and it is this that basically powers us and fuels every
single cell in the body. Cells contain different numbers of mitochondria according to the amount of energy required in that
tissue, so the brain and heart cells, for example, will have a higher
mitochondria count than some other organs. (If you think of
each body cell as being like a car battery, the mitochondria are
the equivalent of the energy cells within this.) Young people have
fit and active mitochondria, but these age as we do, and so as we
get older physical consequences of this process can develop. Some
scientists have recently got very excited about the notion that all
our ageing processes could be slowed or even stopped by preventing mitochondrial damage, but how this is to be achieved is
still in the realms of fantasy.

Even so, there are steps we can take to keep our mitochondria
as fit as possible. It is obvious that a healthy lifestyle is best – don't

smoke, eat fresh food, rest your body, exercise regularly – but there are supplements that may help too. One I have mentioned earlier in this section is CoEnzyme Q_{10}, a key player in optimal energy production. Another is carnitine, a naturally occurring amino acid that seems to work by carrying fat molecules into mitochondria to be converted into energy. This also boosts the production of an enzyme called cytochrome oxidase, which is also needed for effective 'energy making'. With both CoEnzyme Q_{10} and carnitine safe and free of side effects, it would seem sensible to try them if your energy levels appear low or if chronic fatigue is a problem. Most experts recommend doses of 30 milligrams of CoEnzyme Q_{10} and 400–500 milligrams of carnitine, both taken twice daily, but these dosages can be increased during times of great stress.

Mitochondria are the energy factory in our body's cells. These age as we do, but you can boost their performance by using the supplements CoEnzyme Q_{10} and carnitine.

Stretch and flex

Why is the number of flexibility classes increasing so rapidly? Not many years ago these often took the form of a cliquey exercise programme held in small groups, but now thousands of people flock to take part in Pilates, t'ai chi, yoga and many other classes designed to promote flexibility and suppleness. This is partly because it is a little trendy, but also because people enjoy the range of benefits that such exercises offer. Instead of just working one group of muscles, as in, say, weight training, they work many groups at the same time. Posture, balance and co-ordination are improved, all with low-impact techniques. Muscles become strengthened and lengthened without an associated increase in bulk (I know very few women who want to look like Arnold Schwarzenegger) and an emphasis on correct breathing leaves people revitalised rather than exhausted.

So, how to stretch? There are four main techniques. Passive stretching is where exercises are partner-directed, as often occurs at the end of a session, and an example would be a partner or trainer pressing your leg towards your body to stretch your hamstrings. These are helpful in preventing post-exercise muscle fatigue and weakness. Active stretching moves a limb through its full range of motion. Pilates exercises are a good example of this. Static stretches hold muscles in certain positions for up to 30 seconds. Finally, there are 'tense and relax' stretches, or PNF (proprioceptive neuromuscular facilitation), which are probably the most effective way to increase ranges of motion. Here a partner or prop is used to allow muscles to be stretched deeply, contracted and relaxed.

Whatever kind of stretching you practise, remember that you are not going to burn off hundreds of calories in this way. The aim here is to improve muscle tone, suppleness and posture, but if you want to lose weight you will need to add dieting and aerobic exercise to your personal programme. By increasing flexibility you enhance muscle performance, and this benefits the youthful athlete and elderly individual alike.

Always remember:

★ Never do stretching exercises without warming up first.

★ Never try to increase your stretch by repeatedly straining.

★ Hold stretches for 10–30 seconds.

★ Do each stretch at least twice.

★ Tightness is an acceptable feeling when you are stretching, but pain is not.

★ After finishing one set of stretches, move out of position gently and slowly.

Stretching may not have you puffing and panting as some forms of exercise do, but a supple body will help to prevent many musculo-skeletal health problems. Use it as part of an overall programme of fitness allied to a sensible diet and swimming or walking.

Learn to do nothing

You will not find this tip in any medical textbook but there is one activity that I am convinced is healthy for us all but which most of us are extremely bad at – doing absolutely nothing. This was brought home to me recently when I came out of hospital after fairly heavy spinal surgery and was forced to sit or lie about doing very little indeed.

What surprised me was not any frustration I had about my physical condition, but the fact that I was actually having to do nothing instead of rushing around at 100 miles an hour like I normally do. The more I thought about it, the more I realised how foreign the concept of just doing nothing was to me, and how unhealthy that is. However, after several days I realised that resistance was futile and settled back into doing what I should – nothing. By the end of the first week I was beginning to relax and after another fortnight I was practically comatose. I had reached a level of relaxation that was practically foreign to me, yet all I had done was simply stop and do nothing. No health spas, no personal gurus, no change in diet – I simply stopped. I am the same when I go on holiday – not only does it take a week to begin to relax and feel the benefit of being away from work, but by the time the holiday is over I am just starting to enjoy myself.

Of course, I would not recommend such a drastic way of finding time to relax as having an operation, but many of us do – usually of necessity – lead very busy lives and often become used to feeling stressed and frazzled. As a result it can be necessary to deliberately take a step back from what we are doing and make a conscious effort to go down several gears. What we choose to do is up to us – some people garden, some watch football and others simply put their feet up and enjoy doing nothing at all.

A busy lifestyle can leave us little 'quality time' to look after ourselves, but check how often you find yourself saying, 'I should be doing something', and you will probably be surprised. Next time you do, ask yourself, 'Why?', and unless it is crucially important, give yourself a break instead. This is not boredom, but simply switching off for a few minutes and allowing yourself to relax.

Someone who found it difficult to switch off was the playwright George Bernard Shaw. At a performance given by an Italian string quartet, a companion murmured to him, 'These men have been playing together for twelve years.' 'Surely,' came back the reply, 'we have been here longer than that.'

Learn to do nothing. Our bodies and minds need rest and recuperation as much as food and drink. The harder you find it to do this, the more your body may need to.

'The tragedy of old age is not that one is old, but that one is young.'

— Mark Twain

Mind and Body tips

Smile – it could be worse

How many times have you heard yourself say, 'I could do with a good laugh'? Plenty, I expect. For me, this poses no particular problem – I simply take my clothes off and look at myself in the mirror. However, there is more to the subject of humour than may at first meet the eye, and it is no coincidence that in America clowns roam the children's wards and have been shown to reduce those children's need for painkillers simply by cheering them up.

For most of us laughter is occasional rather than frequent, which is a huge shame. As a doctor I suppose I belong to a medical club (along with the other emergency services) where the humour is often dark and tragic – as well as being intensely funny – and helps us to cope with some of the more intense experiences of the working day. As adults we often lose the knack of laughing at the absurdities of life, which I think explains why certain comedians, such as Billy Connolly, are so funny. They do not so much tell jokes as point out humorous things we have all seen but missed the point of.

A good belly laugh can exercise most muscles in our body ('I laughed until I ached'), clear our lungs, increase our circulation and release the natural painkillers endorphins into our bodies.

An American study showed how even the thought of a good laugh can be beneficial. Men were given formal psychological tests two days before, 15 minutes before and immediately after watching their own choice of an hour-long humorous video. Their tension, depression and anger ratings rather surprisingly began to fall two days before they saw the video, showing that looking forward to a laugh can benefit mood and even the immune system. This ties in with a smaller study which indicated that people with heart disease appeared to laugh less (although this is a huge and multi-factorial disease), as do people with smaller social circles and fewer friends.

I always try to use the '3 Rs' of humour to get its maximum benefits. 1. Remind yourself to look for the humorous things in life. 2. Remember the funny thing that has happened. 3. Retell what has happened to someone else. Ask comedians if they have ever had any kind of psychotherapy and most will say, 'Therapy? What do you think I go on stage for?'

I will always remember one elderly man who had requested that his sperm count be tested. I did not think this was appropriate, but after much cajoling from him – and for a quiet life – I agreed and sent him out of my room with the appropriate sample pot. When he reappeared the next day with an empty pot, I sympathised but was stopped by his insisting, 'No, Doc, you don't understand. I went home like you said, and got straight down to it. I tried with my left hand, then with my right. Then the wife tried with her left hand, and then with her right. Finally she tried with her teeth in, and then with her teeth out, but it was useless. We still couldn't get the top off the bloody jar.'

Humour is essential in our difficult world. Make time to laugh, remember what made you chuckle in the first place and tell it to other people to get the benefit a second time.

'You mean sex is good for you as well?'

This was the classic response I got from a patient when I mentioned that an active sex life in their eighth decade was doing them a power of good. When the Creator was dishing out pleasurable activities for man to do, he was certainly cooking with gas that day, because sex has been a driving force throughout all humankind ever since.

If we look beyond the fact that sex, like the need for shelter, food and warmth, is a basic human driving force, it becomes clear that there are a number of reasons why, on grounds of health, it should be encouraged into old age:

★ It can keep you fit. Believe it or not, sexual intercourse can burn off 150 calories every half hour, but this figure obviously varies according to factors such as age, mood, enthusiasm and whether you have just won the lottery. This is better than not burning those calories off, and more enjoyable than going to the gym.

★ Believe it or not, having two orgasms or more per week may actually help men to live longer. At each orgasm the level of the hormone DHEA increases in response to ejaculation and this has a number of effects, including acting as an antidepressant and boosting the immune system – useful for a healthy life.

★ Testosterone and oestrogen levels can be boosted through regular sexual activity. In men, testosterone can be beneficial to the heart and musculo-skeletal system, and in women oestrogen may protect against heart disease.

★ The increase in blood flow through our bodies during sex has the same effects as that which occurs during exercise, and so if this is repeated several times a week fitness can actually increase.

★ After sex, people tend to sleep better and awake feeling more refreshed. Regular sex is also said to help people to handle stress better by acting as a physical release for tension and pressure.

★ Sex can help to reduce chronic pain. Whenever you have sex, the hormone oxytocin is released into the body and this not only helps to trigger orgasm but also causes the release of endorphins – the body's version of morphine. Because of this, headaches, cramps and general aches and pains can be reduced by simply having fun.

★ A decade-long study published in the *British Medical Journal* stated that men who had sex less than once a month had double the death rate of those who had sex at least twice a week. And don't worry if you haven't got a willing partner – it's the number of orgasms that is important here rather than the notches on your bedpost.

There is an interesting caveat to all the above points, though, and one which may make interesting reading to philandering men. If a man is having an affair, his risk of having a heart attack during sex is greater than if he is making love to his wife. There is prob-ably a music-hall gag in there somewhere, but I'm not going to go for it. Joking apart, happiness is not sex, but sex can play a part in happiness, whatever your age.

Sex is one of nature's best ways of keeping fit, relaxed and healthy. Many sexual problems can now be treated, so if you feel there is a problem in your sex life don't be afraid to seek help.

Look on the bright side

Mark Twain famously remarked that he had suffered from many problems in his life, most of which had never happened. I am rather fond of this quotation whenever I am wrestling with an anxiety-provoking thought in the middle of the night, because it reminds me that I have built a whole scenario around absolutely nothing at all since it hasn't happened yet and probably never will. End of worry and back to sleep.

Now this is in fact a form of pessimism, as most pessimists believe in the Eeyore principle, which says that something dreadful is just bound to happen to them despite a complete lack of evidence to support this. Well, believe it or not, pessimism can actually be bad for you – optimists outlive their pessimistic counterparts according to a number of wide-ranging studies, and I suppose there is a simple reason. Pessimists are people who basically blame themselves when something goes wrong, and feel that one simple mistake can blight a life. Bad things await them around every corner and they fully expect to meet these problems every day, yet avoid taking any simple measures to prevent their occurrence. When they do occur – as they do in all our lives – their cycle of pessimism is strengthened and it is no surprise to me that many such people die as a result of violence, suicide or accidents.

In one study from the Mayo clinic in America, the happiest people involved showed a 19% reduction in their risk of death compared with their miserable counterparts, with the pessimists' survival rates being far lower than expected for their age. To look at it more scientifically, happiness and optimism can actually strengthen the immune system to help to fight off disease. You would think there would be no sterner test of this than in HIV-positive patients, but one trial showed that such men who thought their condition could be controlled or at least stabilised had a higher 'helper' T-cell count, and lived an average of nine months longer, than their downbeat equivalents. Similar findings have been reported in breast-cancer patients, and although it is by no means some kind of panacea, a positive mental attitude really can improve your health in general.

Instead of worrying over the classic adage of whether your cup is half full or half empty, just remember that a great many people have no cup at all.

Don't sweat over what hasn't happened yet. Let things roll off your back, and concentrate on what is good rather than on problems, real or imagined.

Get out more

When I was a young boy there was a television programme called *Why Don't You Switch Off Your TV Set and Go and Do Something Less Boring Instead?* My, how we laughed at the irony of the title, though I never actually watched it. First, because it was pretty awful, but also because I had taken the title to heart and was off enjoying myself in other ways. However, in this dreadful question there was in fact a kernel of healthy advice and a good reason why we should resist the temptation to slump in front of our televisions as a way of using our recreational time.

Researchers have found that social activities increase both the quality and length of life and a number of reports have come to the same conclusion. We are social animals and are designed through evolution to interact with one another rather than going through life on our own. This truth is so deeply ingrained in us that we still raise both eyebrows at people who choose to live alone or seek a quiet life in the middle of nowhere.

The exact reason why belonging to a friendly group or doing activities socially together could increase our longevity is not easy to pin down, but more socially active people do seem less likely to smoke cigarettes than loners, as well as eating better quality food, exercising more frequently and going to their doctor for check-ups. Talking to people and friends also gives us the opportunity to receive support in times of need, and to discuss and learn from one another about health issues. I am constantly noticing the numbers of patients – especially women – who come to me with a problem that 'I wouldn't normally have bothered you with, Doctor', but who either have been persuaded to attend by friends or have decided to come anyway after a chat with a social group at a party or other gathering.

Personally, I believe anything that raises people's awareness of health is to be applauded, and social contact can play a major role here. Taken on its own, this can seem a small factor in long-term good health and indeed I suppose it is. However, a strong social network fits in with our essentially gregarious natures and is probably doing us good even while we are out enjoying ourselves.

Get out and do more with family and friends. Socially active individuals appear to lead a healthier lifestyle than their less active and more isolated counterparts.

'If anyone knows a reason why these two people should not marry, sit on it'

Groucho Marx is one of my all-time favourite comedians, not just because of his films but also for his spontaneous and witty responses to comments directed at him. A classic example of this occurred during his stint as a comedian on the American television show *You Bet Your Life*. He was interviewing a lady called Mrs Storey, who had given birth to 22 children. 'I love my husband,' said Mrs Storey very enthusiastically. Quick as a flash, Groucho smiled and said, 'I like my cigar too. But I take it out once in a while!'

Although he would not have known it, the well-loved Mr Storey may have been living longer by being in a happy, long and fruitful marriage. A 20-year study by the University of Warwick found that married men live an average of three years longer than single men, and a number of causes have been postulated as to why this should be so. There may be physiological effects that enhance well-being and so promote longevity, and the lifestyle encouraged within marriage may be generally healthier than that of single men. Another interesting theory is that marriage produces a Darwinian desire to impress the other partner, although observing some of my married male patients with their beer guts and interesting personal habits makes me somewhat sceptical on this point.

For what it is worth, my own belief is that marriage (and by this term I mean a healthy and well-balanced partnership rather than a dysfunctional one that is a marriage in name alone) is healthy on a number of fronts. Wives are often very good at looking after their man on the quiet, taking an increasing interest in what they eat and drink the older they get. Companionship and shared interests add mental stimulation, another healthy benefit, and regular sex is physically beneficial. All these health benefits apply to both husband and wife. Some men still cling to the idea that being married is the same as bigamy – having one wife too many. However, those who are lucky enough to be very happily married may be benefiting in ways we are not even aware of.

A happy marriage appears to be beneficial to both mind and body, adding years to life as well as life to years. These benefits can also accrue when a person marries late or remarries.

Stay busy

If there is one phrase I dread hearing when patients talk to me about retiring, it is the one that goes something like, 'I'm just going to sit and do nothing – it'll be great.' Great it may be, dangerous it certainly is. Retirement is actually a perilous time, and the older we are when we retire, the greater are our chances of becoming sick after stopping work. At the moment it is only the occasional day (and usually a very bad one) when I sit back in my surgery chair and dream of driving a sports car very fast along a sunny road abroad and not having to work, yet retirement approaches us all faster than most of us realise. The key is not to worry about retiring – what fun – but to make sure that you do not view retirement as some kind of antechamber where you spend years waiting for God.

When I ask centenarians and other very old people what the secret of being old is, there is one answer I get that is head and shoulders above all the others – 'I keep busy.' Keeping busy can mean anything from flower arranging to scuba diving to discovering how to use a computer. The nature of the activity is almost immaterial – it is the frame of mind that is so important here. We assume that an 80-year-old woman living by herself must be lonely, yet she may have plenty of positive social interactions with others outside her home. At the same time we think that a 70-year-old man who lives with his son's family cannot be lonely, yet he may spend all day in front of the TV set and shun all social activities. Who is the healthier both mentally and physically?

There are many reasons why keeping busy can be good for you, but the following seem to be particularly important:

★ Busy people tend to have more social interactions than isolated people do, and so have wider social and support networks.

★ Busy people often have a greater sense of self-worth.

★ Busy people are often more physically active than people who choose to spend their time in front of the TV.

★ Busy people feel less old than sedentary people.

★ Busy people often have more muscle mass than other people of their age. If people become inactive as they age, they lose muscle mass and this can lead to frailty, falls and broken hips and bones. Health goes, fitness goes, independence goes.

Busy people enjoy retirement and old age far more than those who believe their best years are behind them. Age really can be a state of mind.

Do a crossword

When we talk about exercise we tend to think about the body. But the brain needs regular exercise too, and there is now evidence that the more the brain is stimulated, the greater the likelihood that longevity will increase in that person. Time and again in my medical practice I see healthy people retiring from busy jobs in their sixties only to find them a shadow of their former selves a year or two later. What has happened in the meantime? Did they suddenly become physically unwell or succumb to an unforeseen illness? Not at all. What has happened is quite simple really – they stopped exercising their brains.

Every time we learn something new we strengthen the connections between our brain cells, as well as causing new connections to occur. This can have a beneficial effect as, in later life, brain cells are lost, since the brain can continue to function normally. When explaining this to patients I sometimes use the analogy of a busy city with only one road going into it. If there is a disaster on that road, everything grinds to a halt, but if there are a dozen roads going into the city, then everything continues to flow reasonably well and the disruption is minimal.

It does not really matter what you choose to do as long as you find it intellectually challenging or exciting. The whole new generation of 'silver surfers' embody this well, since they can spend their free time doing anything they choose on the Internet and use the computer as a tool at the same time, reaping the subsequent benefits to the brain. Crossword puzzles, quizzes, chess matches, reading, courses – it is entirely up to you. The key, though, is to not assume that once you have reached retirement age there is little more that you can usefully do – this is a terrible waste. If you have 20 or 30 years of life left, do you really want to spend those years aimlessly? I think not. Longevity is positively correlated with the level of a person's education and the extent to which that person is still involved with intellectual activities. Use it or lose it.

Mental exercise is just as important as physical exercise and promotes longevity. Never use age as an excuse for not learning or challenging your intellect.

Try meditation

I occasionally write about things that I have no experience of, but which I know would probably be good for me if I tried them. Top of the list is meditation, a subject people often think they know about when in fact they are influenced simply by thoughts of hippies sitting cross-legged chanting. I tend to use that most typical of excuses – I have no time – that prevents people in the West taking up this form of relaxation, but when you look at the possible health benefits you may begin to wonder why more of us don't make time for meditation. It:

★ Alters our brain-wave patterns to slow alpha-type waves that induce mental and physical relaxation.

★ Lowers blood pressure.

★ Relieves stress and depression.

★ May help to lower cholesterol levels.

The word 'meditation' derives from the Latin word for 'to contemplate', but some people tell me that their early experiences were anything but contemplative or restful. The combination of learning to sit completely still and empty the mind of thought was completely beyond them, and it was only practice and perseverance that allowed them to benefit in the long term. This is probably why so many people try it and then give up after a while, disappointed that they have not suddenly turned into stress-free paragons of health. But it is clear from those who have persisted with meditation that the benefits will come if you do likewise.

There are a great many meditation techniques and it probably does not matter which one you practise, since the aim is always the same – to achieve as deep a sense of physical and mental relaxation as possible. Having talked to many exponents, many tell me the essence is to sit still, in a cross-legged posture (or as near as you can get to one) and with a straight back. Focus on your breathing and concentrate exclusively on its rhythmic, slow pattern. Do not expect this to be easy at first, or for your mind to be able to clear itself of clutter instantly. This takes time, since we are all used to rushing around thinking of a hundred different things. Some people prefer to meditate alone, others in groups, but it really does not matter. Stick with it and you have nothing to lose except your stress and your high blood pressure.

Meditation is the ultimate way to relax. Its proven health benefits include lowering blood pressure and preventing depression. Find a type that suits you, and remember that practice really does make perfect here.

Try yoga

It seems that you cannot open a magazine or turn on the TV without seeing some pop star or celebrity espousing the virtues of yoga. However, far from being a new type of healthy activity, it has been practised for at least 5,000 years and is one of the most influential components of Hinduism. The good news is that anyone, of any age, can do it, provided they have a quiet space and a little time.

The aim of yoga is to restore the body and mind to its natural healthy state and it does this using three linked disciplines – meditation, breathing techniques and body movements.

Meditation – the deep quieting of the mind and the elimination of negative thoughts – reduces stress levels and has been shown to lower blood pressure and pulse rates and to improve mental functioning and the ability to cope with stress.

Breathing in yoga concentrates on deep, slow and focused breathing patterns that are usually linked with body movements. This type of breathing differs from the shallow pattern of breathing we tend to use when we are rushing around each day, and promotes greater oxygenation of our body, as well as reducing stress.

Specific yoga movements, or postures, benefit tone and strengthen muscle by improving flexibility, balance and posture, so allowing the release of muscle tension and promoting relaxation. Some yoga advocates go further by saying that correctly performed postures help to clear 'obstructions' in the body and in doing so eliminate toxins and impurities.

There is no denying the sometimes quite remarkable effects yoga can have on people's health. It is not a replacement for medical treatment but, if practised regularly, it does seem to benefit many disorders. These include:

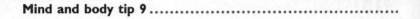

★ depression

★ anxiety

★ insomnia

★ chronic fatigue

★ arthritis

★ stress-related disorders.

The combination of relaxing the brain, breathing correctly and stretching the body is so obvious it makes you wonder why everyone is not practising yoga. Even children can benefit, and as we all seem to experience increasing levels of stress in our daily lives, perhaps this safe way of creating a healthy mind and body will become even more popular.

Yoga is one of the oldest forms of exercise for both mind and body. It can be practised at any age, alone or in groups, and has undoubted health benefits for many people.

Keep a pet

Most mornings I stumble out of bed and begin the daily ritual of walking the dogs as my first task of the day. To be more precise, they walk me while I try to get my higher mental functions to click into gear, but although it often does not seem like it – especially in the dark of winter, lashed by freezing rain – it is probably doing me some good. Apart from the exercise – in my case, walking for miles up hill and down dale watching the dogs disappear out of sight – there are a great many other health benefits available to having a pet, and this need not be restricted to dogs.

Hospices have long recognised that cats and dogs can provide significant help to terminal patients by lowering anxiety levels, promoting relaxation and even reducing the need for strong painkillers. Their presence can decrease feelings of loneliness and isolation as well as helping in the treatment of depression. And, in our cost-conscious times, there can be financial benefits too. An American study published in 1995 found that medication costs dropped from an average of nearly $4 a day to just over $1 in new nursing homes that had both animals and plants as part of their normal environment.

It seems that pets can help us to live longer too. How can this be? It is probably a combination of physical and mental factors. On the physical side, pet owners often appear to have lower levels of both blood pressure and cholesterol than non-owners. Psychologically, pet ownership can promote self-esteem and provide companionship in later years. To return to the American study, the daily living activities of older people who did not own pets deteriorated more rapidly than those who did.

Children gain benefits too, since their cognitive development seems to be enhanced by pet ownership. One study reported that

70% of families surveyed reported an increase in family happiness and fun after acquiring a pet. Family pets may promote nurturing behaviour in children, which can then stay with them into adulthood. Also, the presence of a pet during a childhood illness may decrease the child's stress-related symptoms at that time.

So, should we all be popping down to our nearest pet shop to buy a health-giving rodent, canine or elephant? Of course not – pet ownership is a responsible task and makes various demands, including time, money and motivation. However, if you do own a pet and it is part of your daily routine, this may well be a factor in promoting longevity when taken as one piece of the complex jigsaw that we call good health.

As we grow older, pet ownership can play an increasingly important role in reducing stress, alleviating health problems and warding off loneliness. You may not realise it, but a cat or dog may be better for you than you think.

Swimming – the best exercise of all?

Whenever patients ask me what is the best exercise for them, I almost always tell them: 'Swimming.' As little as an hour and a half per week can make a significant difference to health, and there are a number of reasons why I champion it. The first is that it provides the same aerobic benefits for the heart and lungs as other activities but, unlike, say, jogging, it works *all* the muscles of the body. Also, because the water supports the body, swimming does not put the strain on the joints and musculo-skeletal system that aerobics and running can, and so it rarely leads to injury. I often see runners and gym enthusiasts with injuries they have sustained while exercising, but see surprisingly few such problems in swimmers. Along with physical fitness come psychological benefits, including an increase in well-being and libido and a reduction in stress.

I know what you're going to say, since I've said it myself and my patients do too. 'But I'm too busy to go swimming.' Yet a useful amount of swimming really can take much less time than you think. According to the American Heart Association – and don't forget that swimming is America's most popular recreational health activity – as little as 30 minutes of swimming three times a week will not only improve the condition of your heart and lungs, but will also lower blood pressure, help with weight reduction and decrease total cholesterol levels in the body as part of a balanced exercise and diet programme. If you are able to swim daily, or perhaps four or five times a week, this will bring even greater health benefits.

While researching this book I came across a study published in the journal *Circulation* which proved exactly this point. Four half-hour sessions of swimming a week in a group of out-of-shape, middle-aged businessmen lowered their blood pressure by an average of six points for the systolic and ten points for the diastolic – and it took only ten weeks.

One more point. Swimming usually provides enjoyment, and this can be crucial in keeping it up once the initial enthusiasm has passed. High-intensity exercise programmes often suffer from high drop-out rates because people become frustrated if they cannot meet the standards expected of them. The slower, more comfortable pace of swimming will still keep you healthy, since exercising at 60% of maximum capacity for your age provides as much protection against heart disease as full-speed workouts. Aim for consistency rather than intensity in the pool and you won't go far wrong.

If you are in doubt about which exercise may be best for you, always consider swimming – it can provide the complete package and can be continued into very old age.

Remember to breathe

Of all the important things in life, breathing is right up there with the best of them. During an average day you'll take about 12 breaths per minute at rest, or just over 17,000 in a day. Normally we don't notice our breathing because it is a reflex action, and so we spend much of our time 'shallow breathing' rather than getting the benefit of using our diaphragm muscles. We probably use less than half our lung capacity, which is not good for our long-term health. Breathing properly not only makes us feel generally healthier, but also reduces our levels of stress, strengthens our immune system and improves the quality and quantity of oxygen that is delivered to our cells. Air also keeps the brain active – we need nearly three times more oxygen for our brain than for any other organ, so mental sharpness often comes with better breathing. A good illustration of these health benefits is the fact that regular runners appear to suffer our usual age-related complaints later in life than sedentary people because their breathing patterns are better.

How to breathe then? The key is to breathe from your diaphragm, not your upper chest. At its most extreme, shallow breathing triggers panic attacks in the following way. Upper-chest breathing causes body oxygen levels to fall. This causes a body response and an adrenalin surge. Adrenalin triggers palpitations, anxiety and muscle spasms, with the result that breathing becomes shallower, causing oxygen levels to fall . . . The simplest way of learning to breathe correctly is to:

1. Lie down or sit comfortably and breathe in through your nose. As this happens, push your abdomen (belly) and stomach out. Your chest will continue to expand, so allow your shoulders to go light and expand with it. Count slowly

to five as you are doing this, and don't be tempted to hurry – the slower the better.

2. Hold your breath for a moment, then breathe out slowly through your mouth, counting to five once more. Focus on what you are doing as hard as you can, and be aware of how you are feeling.

3. Repeat this cycle of breathing in and out five times, rest for two minutes and then do it again.

This pattern of breathing is not only good for your long-term health, but is also a quick way to reduce stress. It can be done anywhere – sitting in a traffic jam, before an important interview or during an exam.

I firmly believe that one of the reasons why exercise regimes such as yoga or Pilates are so successful is that they emphasise the importance of focused deep breathing. Luckily, we do not need to roll out the exercise mats to benefit from doing what we were designed to do – breathe.

Being aware of your breathing can be taken to extremes, though. As he lay on his deathbed, a famous nineteenth-century physician gave a medical commentary on his gradual decline. His attendants heard his voice become weaker and weaker until finally he said, 'Pulse – very faint.' A long pause. 'Breathing – stopped.' He spoke no more.

Learn to breathe deeply from your diaphragm. This has many long-term health benefits, especially if practised regularly, and can also be used as a 'stress buster' in a crisis.

Try Pilates

Call me a cynic – and remember that a cynic is simply a realist with experience – but I have become rather used to health fads and exercise crazes coming and going with alarming speed. As long as these do no harm, I'm happy to accept that some people will throw money at anything that promises to give them a new body, a fantastic sex life, endless energy and so on.

However, from time to time something new appears that is actually based on common sense, and a good example is Pilates. Although this system of body toning and fitness has been around for decades, it is only relatively recently that its benefits have become widely known. This unique form of mental and physical conditioning is based on both Western and Eastern disciplines and is increasingly used by sportsmen in the treatment and prevention of injuries. The aim is to achieve precision in muscle control, strength and flexibility, and a great advantage is that it can be done at any age from nine to 90. Although it does little to improve cardiovascular fitness, it will make you feel much suppler and therefore more able to do any other exercise you choose.

One of the reasons I like Pilates is that relaxation is crucial, and this is good for anyone's health. You have to concentrate hard on what you are doing, so the distractions of everyday life melt away, and because your body is deliberately and slowly aligned in the correct anatomical position, there should be little risk of causing any serious damage to it. Movements are co-ordinated and flowing and focus on a strong back, pelvic and abdominal 'centre', which must be created before you move. The best time to exercise is probably in the late afternoon or early evening, when the activities of the day have warmed up your muscles. You need very little equipment, but a clear floor space is essential.

Pilates can help with many common health problems, especially back pain. It can also deal with foot trouble, such as flat feet, by realigning the lower limbs correctly and taking excessive strain off the hip joints. Exercising joints through their normal full range of movements encourages the natural production of synovial fluid, which 'oils' them. Arthritis sufferers are often helped in this way, because the joint is exercised fully without placing it under undue strain. Of all the benefits of Pilates, however, perhaps the most commonly seen is the prevention and treatment of tension headaches, especially if this condition is triggered by poor posture.

Former Wimbledon champion Pat Cash has said that Pilates exercises have been for him some of the most beneficial he has ever tried, but you do not need to be a world champion to get the benefits. However, if you have a problem with your back or are pregnant, it is sensible to take medical advice before starting a new exercise programme such as this. Whether practised individually or in classes, self-taught or coached, Pilates really can offer something for everyone, even in old age.

If you are looking for a system of exercises to promote flexibility and correct posture, Pilates may be for you. It can also benefit your general health in many ways.

To sleep or not to sleep

Looking back to my days as a medical student, I remember with great fondness an event that occurred at the start of a lecture being given by an eminent professor of the time. All those present were hushed as the great man opened his mouth to further enlighten us, when a dishevelled-looking friend of mine came stumbling through the hall doors like a bull in a china shop. Since the professor was not known for his limitless supply of patience, we awaited the kill, only to hear the classic apology, 'Sorry, sir – my eyelids refused to open.' At the time it seemed such a natural thing to hear, and the latecomer was waved to his seat. It was only much later that we heard that the professor had spent the next half hour trying desperately not to roar with laughter and destroy his reputation.

Insomnia is a general term meaning an inability to get refreshing sleep, and my patients seem to suffer from three main types. First, there is transient insomnia, which lasts no more than a few nights. (Lying awake worrying about exams would be a good example here.) Then there is short-term insomnia lasting up to three or four weeks, and finally chronic insomnia, which persists longer than this. At least 10% of the UK's population feel that they have a problem with chronic insomnia and, as a result, suffer from the effects of sleep deprivation.

Although insomnia is frustrating rather than dangerous, its effects can be significant and even prevent survival into old age. Insomniacs have twice as many road accidents as non-insomniacs, and spend around half as much time working or studying, because of their difficulty in sleeping. Serious accidents at work are commoner in people who sleep poorly, and for them simple tasks often become inappropriately difficult to perform.

Certain common causes of insomnia are obvious, but time and

again I find many people do not consider them, which is a shame, since most cases are readily treatable. It must be remembered that tobacco, alcohol and caffeine all disturb sleep in everyone who uses them, including those who are convinced that these have no effect on them. Although alcohol may be thought of as a relaxant, it is actually a cause of heavily fragmented sleep later in the night and should be avoided close to bedtime. Similarly, chronic smoking will disturb sleep, and because caffeine has a long half-life in some people, they may need to be caffeine-free all evening in order to enjoy better sleep.

Routine also appears to be an important factor in many people, since waking at the same time each morning helps the body's natural rhythms, which in turn help the onset of sleep. There is little point in lying in bed desperately willing yourself to fall asleep. This becomes self-defeating, and it is far better to get up and do something until you feel tired once more. Exercise taken during the day may not guarantee refreshing sleep the same night, but it is good to get into the habit of doing some exercise each day, since this often leads to deeper sleep over time. Try not to go to bed either hungry or too full, and do not have the bedroom too warm, since this can cause you to wake in the early hours. View the bedroom as a place for sleeping rather than for watching TV or working, and remember that sex is one of nature's better ways of promoting deep sleep.

Try to avoid resorting to sleeping tablets. Apart from causing a problem of dependence, they do not promote truly restful sleep. If they are used, it should be only in the short term, in order to encourage a change in sleep pattern.

As an interesting aside here, a six-year study published in America's Archives of General Psychiatry looked at sleep as part of cancer prevention. With 1.1 million participants, this is the first large-scale study of sleep to take into account variable factors such as diet, age, smoking and exercise. It found that a group sleeping eight hours each night was more likely to die younger than those sleeping six to seven hours. As the average Briton gets six and a half hours' sleep nightly, we may be healthier than we think.

If you suffer from insomnia, always look for the obvious reasons, including consumption of alcohol, tobacco and caffeine. Also, remember that the amount of sleep we need diminishes with age, and that 'power naps' of up to 40 minutes during the day are an extremely effective way of keeping body and soul together.

Boost your immune system

Certain people I know seem to be completely immune to any kind of illness throughout the year. Questioning them about the elixir of health, I quickly found out that no such thing exists, since their words of wisdom included smoking a lot, drinking a lot, eating all the wrong things and having freezing showers in the middle of winter. We all know of the fine old chap who, on reaching the age of 100, declares it to be due to his daily habit of 60 cigarettes and a bottle of whisky, but most people stay well because they look after their bodies.

The title of this tip is, I admit, rather disingenuous, since I do not think there is any one best way to boost your immune system, just as there is no perfect diet. However, there are a number of important tips which, despite being no more than common sense, are often forgotten. These include:

★ Eat as much fresh food as possible. This is not always easy, but if you can, do it.

★ Try not to get dehydrated.

★ Laugh a lot. Having good old-fashioned fun (and I leave that definition to you) is good for you.

★ Sleep as well as you can. Sleep fires up our immune systems beautifully and helps us to keep our 'killer T-cells' – the ones that assist in fighting off viral infections.

★ Eat yoghurt. Active yoghurt cultures are a form of probiotics, and these work to clean the body in a similar fashion to antibiotics, but in a natural way.

★ Exercise regularly. Any exercise is better than none, but regular exercise is best.

★ Take supplements that may enhance the immune system, such as echinacea, CoEnzyme Q_{10} and ginseng.

★ Learn to relax and watch life go by – the hardest one of the lot!

There is no miraculous way to achieve a healthy immune system, but it's important to realise that although our bodies often forgive us for what we do to them, they never forget. The healthier we can live now, the better it is in the long term.

Live well and live right to boost your immune system. A combination of diet, fresh food, sleep, exercise and supplements is the best start.

'I've been rich and I've been poor, and rich is better'

John Paul Getty, the US oil executive and a man famed for his fabulous wealth, was once asked by a newspaper reporter if it was true that he was worth a billion dollars. Getty thought for a minute or two and then quietly replied, 'I suppose I am. But remember – a billion dollars doesn't go as far as it used to.'

I see many patients who have a similar frame of mind as far as money is concerned. It seems to them that you can never have quite enough money, so most of their energy is spent on accruing more, regardless of the cost to health or happiness. (Most of the richest people I have met in my life were miserable so-and-sos, who, when I pointed this out to them, told me, 'I can afford to be.') Money – or, to be more precise, worrying about money – is a constant source of stress to people, and families fight over this issue more than any other.

Why should money relate to health anyway? Putting it bluntly, unless we lead the life of an ascetic hermit we need money to live. Food, shelter, warmth and clothing are life's essentials, and these cost money. Being unable to afford proper food is a particularly common problem, even in developed countries, as optimal health can never be achieved without a healthy, nutritious diet. But if this and the other basic needs are not met, people can descend into a spiral of stress, depression and physical problems.

Money worries come top of the list of problems in many strained marriages, and the stress they produce is bad for both physical and mental health. Even rich couples argue about their attitudes to money, and I remember one fabulously wealthy couple sitting in front of me quarrelling heatedly about which of them spent more. When they asked me what my advice was, I simply said, 'Give most of your money away to charities of your choice. If you feel you can't do that, prepare to get divorced.' Six months later they were poorer, but only because their divorce lawyers were richer. Ask yourself why money is so important to you. If it is to provide the best you can for you and your family, that's fine. If it is simply to accumulate possessions and the trappings of wealth, think again. There are few things more saddening than watching a rich man trying to buy his way out of his grave. It never works.

Money is strongly linked to self-esteem and self-worth. If you are satisfied with your financial status (few of us are, in truth), you are likely to report stronger feelings of self-belief and satisfaction than those people who are not. The problem here is that many people, influenced relentlessly by the media, believe that happiness can be achieved only through constantly acquiring things, and so enough is never enough. Acquisition becomes an obsession, and inevitably the same applies to the means of feeding this obsession – money. Enough will do – but we all have to decide how much is enough and accept the possible consequences of always chasing more.

Since money provides most of our basic needs, having too little of it is stressful. However, having more and more is not necessarily better, and can bring its own pressures. Don't line your grave with gold.

Make friends

Some people are surprised when I mention that I can count the number of those I call real friends on the fingers of one hand. True, I have hundreds, if not thousands, of acquaintances that I can happily spend time with. We are all different in the number of close friendships we form, but, however many friends we have, we all derive health benefits from friendship itself.

Supportive and encouraging friends help to keep our thinking in line with the real world, as well as bolstering our hope if we are going through illness or trauma, and increased hope is associated with improved immune-system functioning. If we have little friendship in our lives we become lonely and isolated and these are unhealthy feelings in the long term.

One interesting point about friendship – and one that has been said to partly explain why women live longer than men – is that women seem more ready to seek out friends as a response to stress. Females of many species, including humans, often 'tend and befriend' when stressed, protecting their children ('tending') and seeking social contact and support from other females ('befriending'). Women respond to stress by talking more often on the phone than men to family or friends, or by making simple social contacts, such as asking for directions when lost. Men, by contrast, often try to deal with a problem themselves rather than seeking help. This response may include drinking and smoking more, working longer hours than usual and isolating themselves.

Could this be one of the reasons why women live longer than men by an average of seven years? Even if it is not, common sense dictates that friendship has to be good for us in that it reduces social isolation and provides a sounding board for our problems. When allied to other buffers against stress, such as a sense of humour, an optimistic outlook, physical fitness and a sense of faith, friendship is sometimes better for our health than most of the pills I prescribe every day.

Close friends are invaluable and may be actually doing our long-term health a lot of good. Women probably benefit more from friendship than men because of their greater readiness to share their feelings with friends in times of stress and to help others who are stressed.

You really can change

As we get older, we seem to get more set in our ways. This is often because we like what we like and in any case don't feel the need to branch out and try other things as much as we did when we were younger. However, in talking to centenarians, I found that many of them had made significant changes in their lives and felt that this was one of the reasons for their longevity. These changes did not need to be obvious ones, such as stopping smoking or improving a poor diet, but could involve anything different from what they were used to. Examples were learning computer skills or a foreign language, playing a musical instrument, and taking up writing or painting.

I am certain that the common factor here is a readiness to remain stimulated and interested in things. Although I can never prove it, I am sure that the many enduring interests of HM the Queen Mother – especially her passionate love of racing – contributed to her longevity. Many people believe that life after retirement is a simple slowing-down process until death intervenes, which is an attitude that fills me with horror. It is interesting to look at mortality statistics and retirement, since there is a sharp rise in deaths in the twelve months after work ends. I have seen this a number of times in my patients and, on talking to their spouses, I often find that the partner who died seemed to have simply stopped working, sat down and decided to do nothing. This sudden change of pace is dangerous, it seems, and I always advise retiring people to make sure that they have lots of interests lined up to keep them busy at their own pace. Many people who retire at 65 will have two decades or more left – equivalent to half their working life – and although health problems may restrict what can be done, this does not mean that doing nothing is all there is. You can get excitement and satisfaction from projects at any age, and I genuinely believe that our outlook on life influences our long-term health.

When the mother of Hollywood star Cary Grant was in her nineties, she rang him after watching him on television, to reprimand him for letting his hair go so grey. 'It doesn't bother me at all,' he replied. 'Maybe not,' said his mother sternly, 'but it bothers me. It makes me seem so old, and I'm not.'

Ageing is a state of mind for many people. Don't allow yourself to think that growing older means that you cannot try something new. You can, and you will feel younger for it.

Listen to music

For me, music is one of the great joys in life. Whether we enjoy a classical diet or the latest chart hit, or both, music affects us all. Some two and a half thousand years ago scholars believed that music could cleanse the body, and before that people used chanting and primitive music as a means of communicating with the spirit world and helping the healing process. These days we use the term 'music therapy', but the underlying principle has not changed one jot – music is good for you. It can promote relaxation and reduce insomnia, soothe infants and disturbed children, and help in treating depression.

Doctors working with the elderly in hospitals and care homes have reported that patients who listen regularly to music eat and sleep better, require less medication, quarrel less and seem generally more contented. I sometimes see this in my role as a prison doctor. Young men deprived of their favourite music for long periods become much less aggressive if this pleasure is restored to them.

Music has also been shown to have a perceptible effect on brain function. It can improve the mobility of patients with Parkinson's disease or who have suffered from a stroke, and help with both long-term and short-term memory problems. In the stressed or anxious person, soothing music lowers blood pressure and reduces the heart rate, as well as lessening muscle tension. One of the possible reasons for this was suggested by a recent study on a group of male patients with Alzheimer's disease. Blood tests taken at both the start and the end of a four-week course of music therapy showed a significant increase in the men's levels of melatonin over this time, and this increase continued for some weeks after the therapy ended. Melatonin is thought to be crucial in how the body's natural clock works, and, if this is so, it affects sleep and relaxation patterns. Levels of other body chemicals, such as epinephrine and norepinephrine, also increased significantly during the sessions but returned to pre-therapy levels six weeks afterwards.

Dentists are now using low-toned, monotonous music to alleviate the anxiety many people have about visiting them. Music of this kind appears to reduce patients' emotional tension, but this is hardly surprising because we have known for a very long time how well music can relax people.

Whatever type of music you prefer, if it makes you feel good, enjoy it. However, quiet or soothing music does appear to be the best for helping us to relax. There is an interesting link here with driving. Drivers who prefer loud and fast music have faster pulse rates, drive faster and take more risks than those who listen to quiet or classical music when on the road. Since our roads are not the most relaxing of places at the best of times, it seems sensible to avoid putting petrol on this particular fire.

One night in Vienna, the Duke of Wellington was forced to sit through a performance of Beethoven's *Battle of Victoria*, then also called *Wellington's Victory*. After it had finished, a Russian diplomat asked him if it was anything like the real thing. 'By God, no,' he said. 'If it had been anything like that, I would have run away myself.'

It really does seem that music can touch the hardest soul.

Music relaxes us, helps us to cope with sadness and can improve the quality of our lives. Pick soothing music for the best results.

Your best is good enough

I leave the last words in this book to a patient I knew some years ago. He had served in the Navy during both world wars and whenever I visited him I always used to enjoy listening to his tales of combat. As a young boy during the Great War, he had been a gunner's assistant on a warship and had witnessed many things no young man should see. Over two decades later he patrolled the Atlantic, chasing U-boats, and survived being torpedoed, shot and left for dead. A hard man indeed, but you would never have known it from his manner, which was friendly, placid and utterly charming. Shortly before his death at the age of 98, I asked him what the secret of his long life was and received an interesting reply. 'Doc,' he said, 'I learnt from an early age that my best was good enough. I've been bombed, torpedoed, shot, sworn at and told I was useless more times than I care to remember, but I always knew that I was doing my absolute level best in whatever I did. Knowing that helped me through it all, even when I thought I was a goner, because it really puts everything into perspective.'

I mulled this over until the next time I saw him – which turned out to be the last – and we discussed the subject further. He had realised long ago that if he did not have a sense of self-worth and belief in himself, then no one would, and this proved to be a constant source of help whenever he experienced severe stress in his life. Although not a religious man, he had, during his extensive travels, come across a saying that he had always remembered, and as I write this it comes back to me. It was from the *Bhagavad Gita*, a cornerstone of Hinduism, and said, 'Once you have realised the essential immortality that is the birthright of every human being, then death is no more traumatic than taking off an old coat.' What better way to finish?

Doing your best, and knowing in your heart that you can do no better, can be a source of great comfort during stressful times. Your best is good enough.

Index